SUBSTANCE ABUSE ASSESSMENT, INTERVENTIONS AND TREATMENT

RECOVERY-ORIENTED SYSTEMS OF CARE FOR INDIVIDUALS WITH SUBSTANCE USE PROBLEMS

ELEMENTS, GUIDANCE AND RESOURCES

Substance Abuse Assessment, Interventions and Treatment

Additional books in this series can be found on Nova's website under the Series tab.

Additional E-books in this series can be found on Nova's website under the E-book tab.

SUBSTANCE ABUSE ASSESSMENT, INTERVENTIONS AND TREATMENT

RECOVERY-ORIENTED SYSTEMS OF CARE FOR INDIVIDUALS WITH SUBSTANCE USE PROBLEMS

ELEMENTS, GUIDANCE AND RESOURCES

JONAH EDELMAN
EDITOR

nova publishers
New York

For permission to use material from this book please contact us:
Telephone 631-231-7269; Fax 631-231-8175
Web Site: http://www.novapublishers.com

Library of Congress Cataloging-in-Publication Data

ISBN: 978-1-62808-648-5

Published by Nova Science Publishers, Inc. † New York

CONTENTS

PREFACE

This book reviews the research related to the 12 guiding principles of recovery and the 17 elements of recovery-oriented systems of care developed through the National Summit on Recovery. It also offers an appraisal of scientific literature discussing the recovery-oriented systems of care conceptual framework and literature on recovery-oriented service and systems implementation.

Chapter 1 – The concept of recovery lies at the core of the Substance Abuse and Mental Health Services Administration's (SAMHSA's) mission, and fostering the development of recovery-oriented systems of care and services is a Center for Substance Abuse Treatment (CSAT) priority. In support of that commitment, in 2005, SAMHSA's CSAT convened a National Summit on Recovery. Participants at the Summit represented a broad group of stakeholders, policymakers, advocates, consumers, clinicians, and administrators from diverse ethnic and professional backgrounds. Although the substance use problems and disorders treatment and recovery field has discussed and lived recovery for decades, the Summit represented the first broad-based national effort to reach a definition of recovery and a common understanding of the guiding principles of recovery and the elements of recovery-oriented systems of care.

Through a multistage process, key stakeholders formulated guiding principles of recovery and key elements of recovery-oriented systems of care. Summit participants then further refined the guiding principles and key elements in response to two questions: 1) What principles of recovery should guide the field in the future? and 2) What ideas could help make the field more recovery oriented?

A working definition of recovery, 12 guiding principles of recovery, and 17 elements of recovery-oriented systems of care emerged from the Summit process; these are subsequently defined in this paper and in the *National Summit on Recovery: Conference Report*. These principles and elements can now provide a philosophical and conceptual framework to guide SAMHSA/CSAT and other stakeholder groups and offer a shared language for dialog.

Summit participants agreed on the following working definition of recovery:

> Recovery from alcohol and drug problems is a process of change through which an individual achieves abstinence and improved health, wellness, and quality of life.

The guiding principles that emerged from the Summit are broad and overarching. They are intended to give general direction to SAMHSA/CSAT and other stakeholder groups as the treatment and recovery field moves toward operationalizing recovery-oriented systems of care and developing core measures, promising approaches, and evidence-based practices. The principles also helped Summit participants define the recovery-oriented elements and guided recommendations for the field.

Following are the 12 guiding principles identified by participants (defined in this paper):

- There are many pathways to recovery.
- Recovery is self-directed and empowering.
- Recovery involves a personal recognition of the need for change and transformation.
- Recovery is holistic.
- Recovery has cultural dimensions.
- Recovery exists on a continuum of improved health and wellness.
- Recovery emerges from hope and gratitude.
- Recovery involves a process of healing and self-redefinition.
- Recovery involves addressing discrimination and transcending shame and stigma.
- Recovery is supported by peers and allies.
- Recovery involves (re)joining and (re)building a life in the community.
- Recovery is a reality.

Participants at the Summit agreed that recovery-oriented systems of care are as complex and dynamic as the process of recovery itself. They are designed to support individuals seeking to overcome substance use problems and disorders across their lifespan. Participants at the Summit declared, "There will be no wrong door to recovery" and also recognized that recovery-oriented systems of care need to provide "genuine, free and independent choice" among an array of treatment and recovery support options. Services should optimally be provided in flexible, unbundled packages that evolve over time to meet the changing needs of recovering individuals. Individuals should also be able to access a comprehensive array of services that are fully coordinated to provide support to individuals throughout their unique journeys to sustained recovery.

Summit participants identified the following 17 elements of recovery-oriented systems of care and services (defined in this paper):

- Person-centered;
- Inclusive of family and other ally involvement;
- Individualized and comprehensive services across the lifespan;
- Systems anchored in the community;
- Continuity of care;
- Partnership-consultant relationships;
- Strength-based;
- Culturally responsive;
- Responsiveness to personal belief systems;
- Commitment to peer recovery support services;
- Inclusion of the voices and experiences of recovering individuals and their families;
- Integrated services;
- System-wide education and training;

- Ongoing monitoring and outreach;
- Outcomes driven;
- Research based; and
- Adequately and flexibly financed.

Work conducted after the Summit defined recovery-oriented systems of care as networks of organizations, agencies, and community members that coordinate a wide spectrum of services to prevent, intervene in, and treat substance use problems and disorders. Figure 1 illustrates the components of the recovery-oriented systems of care framework.

Chapter 2 – This white paper has been prepared as a resource for States, communities, and organizations planning for, embarking on, or well into systems-change efforts intended to develop, sustain, or enhance components of recovery-oriented systems of care. While States, communities, and organizations each face unique challenges and opportunities, the lessons learned by those that have already begun this process can serve as an invaluable resource to other States and communities, offering not a template for action but a menu of options and strategies for readers' consideration. This paper is intended to offer snapshots of promising approaches and is designed to serve as a starting point for discussion.

Using the principles and elements as a point of reference, this document will provide a brief overview of CSAT's Access to Recovery (ATR) program and will describe the activities and operations of three States that have taken steps toward the development of recovery-oriented systems of care through ATR grants: Connecticut, Washington, and Wisconsin.

Despite their varying historical, political, and service system contexts, the projects highlighted in this paper provide useful examples of strategies that might be applicable to other States and communities. Each reflects an ongoing systems improvement philosophy that is an essential component of the endeavor to create recovery-oriented systems of care. None provides a complete template or roadmap, since each State and community is unique, and since in the development of recovery-oriented systems of care one seeks not a static end point, but rather a process of continuous systems and services improvement.

These brief case studies are intended to highlight the unique features of each of the three ATR projects, identifying innovative strategies, approaches, and practices that might be helpful to other States and communities as they plan for or implement recovery-oriented approaches.

Chapter 3 – This white paper has been developed as a resource for States, organizations, and communities embarking on systems-change efforts to develop recovery-oriented system. Each State, local government, community, and organization encounters a unique set of opportunities and challenges when it commits to developing recovery-oriented systems of care. Nonetheless, there are many broadly applicable lessons that can be drawn from the experiences of other States and communities.

Developing and implementing recovery-oriented systems of care are rewarding, difficult, and complex processes. This process is relatively new to the addictions treatment and recovery field, and minimal information is available to guide States, communities, and organizations wishing to develop recovery-oriented systems of care. The case studies presented in this document provide examples of recovery-oriented approaches at various stages of development. By providing a range of examples, States and communities can explore approaches best suited to their circumstances. None provides a complete template or roadmap, since each State and community is unique, and since the development of recovery-oriented systems of care is a continuous process of systems and services improvement. Ultimately, each State, organization, and community will develop recovery-oriented systems of care based on individual needs and strengths.

Using the principles and elements as the framework, this white paper will highlight the activities and operations of two statewide systems and one city system that have taken steps toward the development of recovery-oriented systems of care. It will present case studies highlighting work under way in Arizona, Michigan, and the City of Philadelphia. The case studies will describe the following:

- Approaches to systems change;
- Systems and program models;
- Funding mechanisms;
- Challenges encountered, including workforce and training needs, regulatory and other systems barriers, and reluctance to change among key stakeholder groups;
- Research used to inform the approach; and
- Motivating factors and other elements critical to the implementation of recovery-oriented systems of care.

Chapter 4 – This white paper has been developed as a resource for States, organizations, and communities embarking on or strengthening systems change efforts to develop recovery-oriented systems of care. Each State, organization, and community will create a unique design and implementation strategy for recovery-oriented systems of care. The lessons learned by several organizations that have already begun this process are captured in this paper and can serve as an invaluable resource throughout the design and implementation phase.

Developing and implementing recovery-oriented systems of care are a rewarding, difficult and complex process. This process is relatively new to the addictions treatment and recovery field and minimal information is available to guide States, communities, and organizations wishing to develop recovery-oriented systems of care. The case studies presented in this document provide examples, of recovery-oriented approaches within several communities/settings for diverse populations. By providing a range of examples, States and communities can explore approaches best suited to their circumstance. None provides a complete template or roadmap, since each State and community is unique, and since the development of recovery-oriented systems of care is a continuous process of systems and services improvement.

Using the principles and elements as the framework, this white paper will highlight the activities and operations of provider organizations that have taken steps toward the development of such systems. This paper will present four case studies describing:

- The approach used;
- Funding mechanisms used or developed that support the recovery-oriented system;
- Workforce and training issues encountered;
- Research used to inform the structure and programmatic requirements;
- Motivating factors contributing to systems change;
- Challenges or barriers to systems-change efforts; and

- Other elements critical to each agency's implementation of a recovery-oriented system of care.

Agencies used as case studies are Fayette Companies (Peoria, Illinois), and the Behavioral Health Recovery Management Project; White Bison, Inc. and the Wellbriety Movement; the Sheridan Correctional Center Drug Treatment Prison and Re-entry Program and TASC Illinois' role in the project; and the Citizens Planning and Housing Association (CPHA) of Baltimore, Maryland, and their efforts to expand supportive housing in Baltimore.

Chapter 5 – Are you looking for resources on resiliency and recovery-oriented systems of care (ROSC)? Further, have you been reading the headlines concerning national health care reform and wondering how it will impact programs and services within a ROSC? This guide, which contains information from the Substance Abuse and Mental Health Services Administration (SAMHSA), and your colleagues around the country, will assist you with answers to these questions. State and local policy makers responsible for substance use programming, as well as providers of treatment and recovery support services, can look to this guide for information to enhance prevention, treatment, and recovery services as the changes in health care evolve in their communities.

The purpose of this resource guide is to share an overview of ROSC and illustrate how these systems are an integral part of the new health care environment. This guide will align the tenets of health care reform to the benefits, framework, and history of ROSC, and the steps for planning and implementing ROSC. Following each section of the guide's narrative, you will find websites to direct you to specific resources that will assist you in conceptualizing and developing ROSC. The resources in this guide include research studies, white papers, conference presentations, manuals, practice guides, check lists, regulations and a number of other documents that have been prepared in response to the need for systems reform.

The establishment of ROSC is a relatively new concept in the substance use disorder field. The structure of ROSC will likely evolve as these systems mature and are evaluated. However, as States and communities are creating and implementing ROSC, they can learn from one another. At the same time that they are developing ROSC, they must also consider the changes that are occurring as a result of health care reform. Some policy makers and providers have begun to assess their community strengths and needs in this regard and formulate ROSC plans that are compatible with the tenets of national health care reform. The authors hope this resource guide will assist with that process.

One of the most important elements of national health care reform is the expansion of coverage for those with substance use and mental health disorders. The law also requires 'parity' or that group health insurance plans that provide coverage for mental health and substance use disorders be equal to coverage provided for other medical and surgical benefits. These sweeping changes form the foundation for the new health care environment. Ingrained in health care reform is a public health model that supports ROSC through its vision of prevention, screening and early intervention, treatment, and recovery, integrated with primary health care. Complex developments that include new benefit packages and financing strategies, greater use of technology, promotion of evidence-based practices, and the very important linkage with primary care all present opportunities and challenges that will be addressed in months and years to come. For this reason, this resource guide will be a very fluid product. As information on new initiatives and findings becomes available, it will be incorporated into the resource guide to further illuminate this new environment.

The goal of this guide is to arm you with sufficient information to leverage resources that will create the most favorable outcomes for individuals, families and communities.

In: Recovery-Oriented Systems of Care for Individuals … ISBN: 978-1-62808-648-5
Editor: Jonah Edelman

Chapter 1

GUIDING PRINCIPLES AND ELEMENTS OF RECOVERY-ORIENTED SYSTEMS OF CARE: WHAT DO WE KNOW FROM THE RESEARCH?*

Cori Kautz Sheedy and Melanie Whitter

1. BACKGROUND

The concept of recovery lies at the core of the Substance Abuse and Mental Health Services Administration's (SAMHSA's) mission, and fostering the development of recovery-oriented systems of care and services is a Center for Substance Abuse Treatment (CSAT) priority. In support of that commitment, in 2005, SAMHSA's CSAT convened a National Summit on Recovery. Participants at the Summit represented a broad group of stakeholders, policymakers, advocates, consumers, clinicians, and administrators from diverse ethnic and professional backgrounds. Although the substance use problems and disorders treatment and recovery field has discussed and lived recovery for decades, the Summit represented the first broad-based national effort to reach a definition of recovery and a common understanding of the guiding principles of recovery and the elements of recovery-oriented systems of care.

Through a multistage process, key stakeholders formulated guiding principles of recovery and key elements of recovery-oriented systems of care. Summit participants then further refined the guiding principles and key elements in response to two questions: 1) What principles of recovery should guide the field in the future? and 2) What ideas could help make the field more recovery oriented?

A working definition of recovery, 12 guiding principles of recovery, and 17 elements of recovery-oriented systems of care emerged from the Summit process; these are subsequently defined in this paper and in the *National Summit on Recovery: Conference Report*. [1] These principles and elements can now provide a philosophical and conceptual framework to guide SAMHSA/CSAT and other stakeholder groups and offer a shared language for dialog.

---

* This is an edited, reformatted and augmented version of the Substance Abuse and Mental Health Services Administration, Center for Substance Abuse Treatment, dated August 2009.

Summit participants agreed on the following working definition of recovery:

Recovery from alcohol and drug problems is a process of change through which an individual achieves abstinence and improved health, wellness, and quality of life.

The guiding principles that emerged from the Summit are broad and overarching. They are intended to give general direction to SAMHSA/CSAT and other stakeholder groups as the treatment and recovery field moves toward operationalizing recovery-oriented systems of care and developing core measures, promising approaches, and evidence-based practices. The principles also helped Summit participants define the recovery-oriented elements and guided recommendations for the field.

Following are the 12 guiding principles identified by participants (defined in this paper):

- There are many pathways to recovery.
- Recovery is self-directed and empowering.
- Recovery involves a personal recognition of the need for change and transformation.
- Recovery is holistic.
- Recovery has cultural dimensions.
- Recovery exists on a continuum of improved health and wellness.
- Recovery emerges from hope and gratitude.
- Recovery involves a process of healing and self-redefinition.
- Recovery involves addressing discrimination and transcending shame and stigma.
- Recovery is supported by peers and allies.
- Recovery involves (re)joining and (re)building a life in the community.
- Recovery is a reality.

Participants at the Summit agreed that recovery-oriented systems of care are as complex and dynamic as the process of recovery itself. They are designed to support individuals seeking to overcome substance use problems and disorders across their lifespan. Participants at the Summit declared, "There will be no wrong door to recovery" and also recognized that recovery-oriented systems of care need to provide "genuine, free and independent choice" among an array of treatment and recovery support options. Services should optimally be provided in flexible, unbundled packages that evolve over time to meet the changing needs of recovering individuals. Individuals should also be able to access a comprehensive array of services that are fully coordinated to provide support to individuals throughout their unique journeys to sustained recovery.

Summit participants identified the following 17 elements of recovery-oriented systems of care and services (defined in this paper):

- Person-centered;
- Inclusive of family and other ally involvement;
- Individualized and comprehensive services across the lifespan;
- Systems anchored in the community;
- Continuity of care;

- Partnership-consultant relationships;
- Strength-based;
- Culturally responsive;
- Responsiveness to personal belief systems;
- Commitment to peer recovery support services;
- Inclusion of the voices and experiences of recovering individuals and their families;
- Integrated services;
- System-wide education and training;
- Ongoing monitoring and outreach;
- Outcomes driven;
- Research based; and
- Adequately and flexibly financed.

Work conducted after the Summit defined recovery-oriented systems of care as networks of organizations, agencies, and community members that coordinate a wide spectrum of services to prevent, intervene in, and treat substance use problems and disorders. Figure 1 illustrates the components of the recovery-oriented systems of care framework.

2. Purpose Statement

The purpose of this white paper is to review the research related to the 12 guiding principles of recovery and the 17 elements of recovery-oriented systems of care developed through the National Summit on Recovery. It also offers an appraisal of scientific literature discussing the recovery-oriented systems of care conceptual framework and literature on recovery-oriented service and systems implementation.

Policymakers, providers, practitioners, researchers, recovery support staff, and others interested in the concepts of recovery and recovery-oriented systems of care and services frequently seek data to inform policy development, planning, and program and systems development. This white paper has been prepared as a resource to those seeking information on the research related to recovery.

States, communities, and organizations across the nation are developing and implementing recovery-oriented services and systems. In this paper, they will find evidence that supports and validates services and systems improvements based on recovery-oriented approaches.

Finally, this paper establishes a baseline of existing research upon which the treatment and recovery field can continue to build an understanding of recovery and recovery-oriented systems of care. This paper also identifies areas in the recovery research where additional data are needed.

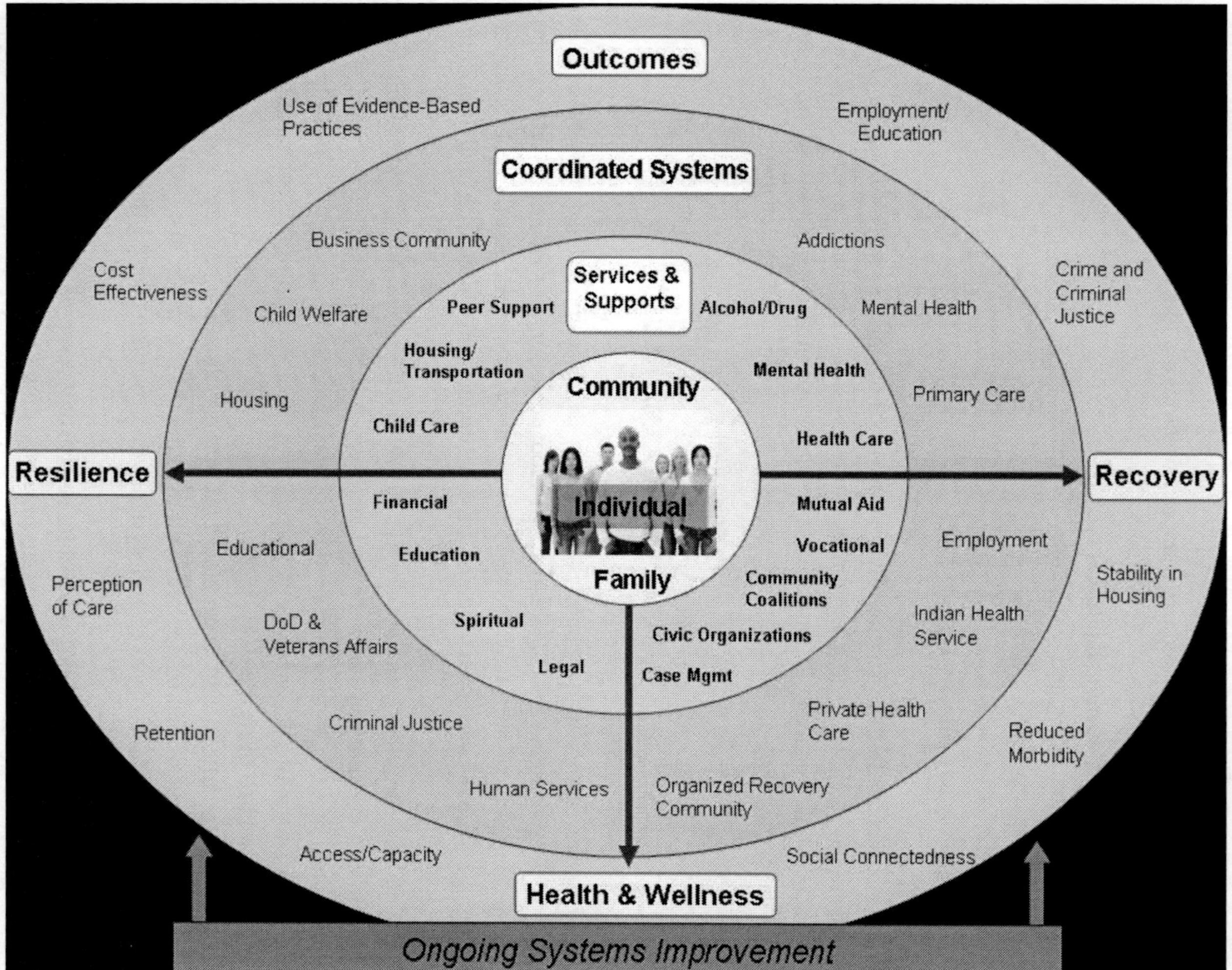

Figure 1. Conceptual Framework of a Recovery-Oriented System of Care.

3. Methodology

Studies included in this paper were identified by searches of electronic bibliographic databases (PsychINFO, PubMed) as well as citations in published studies. Using keywords and established selection criteria related to the principles and systems elements, we conducted a computerized search of health, addictions, financial, and trade journals and newsletters. Many relevant studies were identified. This paper includes a review of research related to recovery-oriented systems of care and services for addiction published in peer-reviewed journals, books, and government publications within the past 20 years, with a focus on the last 10 years.

4. Research Supporting the Conceptual Framework of Recovery-Oriented Systems of Care

Recovery has been called the "organizing construct" for the addictions field.[2] Recently, a conceptual framework that describes and coordinates the delivery of care for individuals with substance use problems and disorders has begun to emerge. Recovery-oriented systems of care are networks of organizations, agencies, and community members that coordinate a wide spectrum of services to prevent, intervene in, and treat substance use problems and disorders. Although States and communities are implementing a variety of services and activities to create recovery-oriented systems, there is minimal research in peer-reviewed journals that examines the framework and the effectiveness and outcomes of this framework. Research is beginning to emerge within the mental health and addictions field related to the recovery-oriented systems of care framework, but the literature is scant. Systems of care research in the addictions field, although conducted within a treatment construct, provides helpful systems information. This section outlines research from the addictions and mental health fields supporting the recovery-oriented systems of care framework, supplemented by research on a systems of care approach within a treatment construct.

In a 2005 article in the *Psychiatric Rehabilitation Journal*, O'Connell, Tondora, Croog, Evans, and Davidson [3] conducted a comprehensive review of the literature on mental illness and addictions recovery that identified the elements of a recovery-oriented environment. According to the authors, a recovery-oriented environment is one that:

- Encourages individuality;
- Promotes accurate and positive portrayals of psychiatric disability while fighting discrimination;
- Focuses on strengths;
- Uses a language of hope and possibility;
- Offers a variety of options for treatment, rehabilitation, and support;
- Supports risk-taking, even when failure is a possibility;
- Actively involves service users, family members, and other natural supports in the development and implementation of programs and services;
- Encourages user participation in advocacy activities;
- Helps develop connections with communities; and

- Helps people develop valued social roles, interests and hobbies, and other meaningful activities.

Gagne, White, and Anthony in a 2007 article in the *Psychiatric Rehabilitation Journal* describe the recovery vision and the values of recovery-oriented care that intersect the addiction and mental health fields:[4]

- Recovery is a personal and individualized process of growth that unfolds along a continuum, and there are multiple pathways to recovery.
- People in recovery are active agents of change in their lives and not passive recipients of services.
- People in recovery from mental illness and/or addiction disorders often note the important role of family and peer support in making the difference in their recovery.
- The values of recovery-oriented mental health and addictions systems are based on the recognition that each person is the agent of his or her own recovery and all services can be organized to support recovery. Person-centered services offer choice, honor each person's potential for growth, focus on a person's strengths, and attend to the overall health and wellness of a person with mental illness and/or addiction.

The authors conclude their discussion by presenting a synopsis of where the mental health and addictions fields concur on how to redesign the systems to assist people in their recovery from mental illness and/or addiction (some are extracted here). According to the authors, recovery should serve as the organizing construct for service provision and for systems improvement.

Additionally, to overcome the limitations of the current acute care model for delivering treatment services, it should be shifted to a community model, where recovery-oriented services are provided in communities, in specific environments of need, and be provided by professionals, family members, and peers. Services are structured to address the long-term and complex needs of people living with addiction and mental health issues. Moreover, to create and operate a recovery-oriented system it should include:

- Principles, e.g., multiple pathways to recovery, recovery is supported by peers, and recovery is non-linear;
- Values, e.g., person-centered services, client choice and, focus on health and wellness;
- Service strategies, e.g., treatment, post-treatment monitoring, early re-intervention, and community support; and
- Essential strategies, e.g., treatment, peer and community support, legal aid, basic support and family formation.[5]

Substance use problems and disorders are preventable and treatable chronic conditions. One aspect of providing recovery-oriented services is the shift from acute care methods to the broader adoption of chronic care strategies throughout the systems of care. Multiple articles have been published in which researchers provide a discussion of the chronic care conceptual framework and the effectiveness of addictions treatment.[6-27] Research in the addictions field uses the treatment system as its organizing construct. Within the recovery-oriented systems of care framework, although the treatment system is central, it is but one of multiple systems. To illustrate this point, research suggests that the service systems that support the initiation of recovery may be different from those that sustain recovery.[28-30]

The life course perspective on drug use is a conceptual framework for understanding drug use trajectories. This framework classifies varying drug use trajectories, identif[ies] critical events and factors contributing to the persistence or change in drug use, analytically order[s] events that occur during the lifespan, and determin[es] contributory relationships".[31, p.515] Hser, Longshore, and Anglin (2007), in presenting the life course perspective on drug use, discuss the evidence demonstrating the multiple service systems that drug users often come in contact with, including drug treatment, criminal justice, mental health, welfare, and primary health. They further state that the interactions with the varied social services system can "trigger turning points" for some individuals and aid in recovery.[32] Turning points are changes in an existing life pathway initiated earlier in one's life and can be positive (e.g., cohesive marriage, meaningful work) or negative (e.g., incarceration, heavy drinking or drug use). The authors' framework incorporates the "patterns or trajectories of drug use across individuals' lives and the ways in which the patterns are shaped by a broader historical context and social structures." [33,p.517]

Babor, Stenius, and Romelsjo (2008) describe elements of a public health approach and conceptual model for the delivery of services and the service systems for people with substance use problems and disorders.[34] The authors primarily focus on the importance of treatment as the organizing construct of the service systems. The model includes specialized services for alcohol and drug dependence as well as medical care and social welfare services that interact with and complement specialized alcohol and drug services.[35] The model also includes the mediators (treatment policies) and moderators contributing to successful outcomes.

The model (Figure 2) outlines the structural resources and qualities of alcohol and drug treatment systems and includes the policy determinants and the population impact of treatment systems. The policy determinants include authoritative decisions made by governmental agencies and legislative policies, regulatory and allocative policies, treatment policies, and system qualities.

In this model:[36]

- Treatment policies are authoritative decisions made by governmental agencies that affect the planning, financing, and monitoring of drug and alcohol services, as well as the development of a professional workforce to operate them.
- Regulatory and allocative policies are major determinants of the structural resources available to treat persons with substance use problems and disorders, including the number of facilities, the types of programs (e.g., detoxification, methadone maintenance, therapeutic communities), the settings where programs operate (e.g., hospitals, social service agencies, specialized drug and alcohol facilities) and the personnel who work there (e.g., drug and alcohol counselors, social workers, psychiatrists, psychologists).

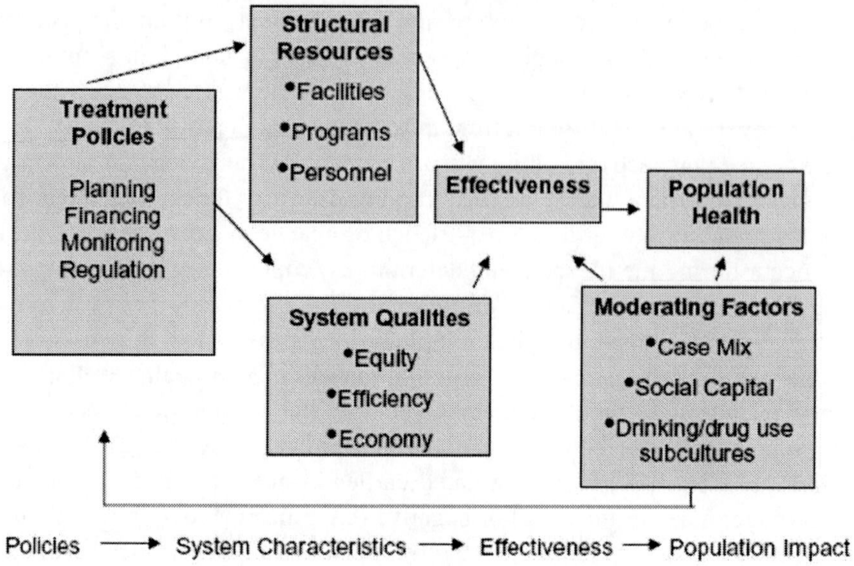

Figure 2. Conceptual Model of Population Impact of Treatment Systems.

- Treatment policies may also affect system qualities, specifying not only where services are located, but also how they are organized and integrated. System qualities include equity (the extent to which services are equally available and accessible to all population groups), efficiency (the most appropriate mix of services), and economy (the most cost-effective services).

As demonstrated by Babor et al., individuals receive alcohol and drug services from a variety of systems, including the specialized alcohol and drug service system; the medical, psychiatric, criminal justice, and social services systems; mutual aid groups; and voluntary organizations. [37] Individuals also receive informal support provided by family and friends, churches and religious organizations, workplace programs, and impaired drivers programs. There are linkages and connections between these formal and informal systems and, depending on the structural resources and system qualities, these sectors will be more or less integrated with specialized treatment and will assume a greater or lesser amount of the responsibility for managing persons with substance use problems and disorders. The authors present an interesting conceptual framework for providing addictions treatment services from a systems perspective.[38] This framework can contribute to the development of the broader recovery-oriented systems of care framework that focuses on providing services throughout the continuum of care and promotes and sustains individual and community recovery.

Minkoff and Cline (2004) present four characteristics of the comprehensive, continuous, integrated systems of care model for organizing services for individuals with co-occurring psychiatric and substance use problems and disorders and the eight principles of treatment for this model.[39] The model's four characteristics are as follows:

1. *System level of change*: The model is implemented into the entire system of care, not only for individual programs or training initiatives.

2. *Efficient use of existing resources*: The model is implemented within the context of current service resources, but emphasizes strategies between each program's requirements and environments.
3. *Incorporation of best practices*: The model is recognized by SAMHSA as a best practice for implementation for those with co-occurring psychiatric and substance disorders.
4. *Integrated treatment philosophy*: The model utilizes a common language for both the mental health and addictions fields.

Minkoff and Cline outline the eight research-and consensus-derived principles that guide the implementation of the model of care and the approach for implementing the complex multilayered system model.[40] The implementation of the model includes the following steps, which the authors detail:

1. Integrated system planning process;
2. Formal consensus on the model;
3. Formal consensus on funding the model;
4. Identification of priority populations and locus of responsibility for each;
5. Development and implementation of program standards;
6. Structures for intersystem and interprogram care coordination;
7. Development and implementation of practice guidelines;
8. Facilitation of identification, welcoming, and accessibility;
9. Implementation of continuous integrated treatment;
10. Development of basic dual diagnosis–capable competencies for all clinicians;
11. Implementation of a system-wide training plan; and
12. Development of a plan for a comprehensive program array.

There is a sizable amount of literature on recovery as the focus of recovery-oriented systems of care in the mental health field. Starting in the early 1990s, the mental health field focused on the process of recovery to guide decisions related to the mental health system. A recovery mental health model puts the locus of control and decision-making in the hands of the person who has the mental health condition.[41-43] "Recovery is pushing systems, as well as providers, to see beyond the diagnostic and categorical services, to treating the individual consumer and his/her multiple needs. The [recovery] vision … is of an external system that reflects the internal reality of its consumers."[44,p.318]

Anthony (1993, 2000) describes the recovery vision and the community support system perspective that provided a framework and essential services of a recovery-oriented systems of care for mental health disorders.[45,46] The author's latest work outlines the relevant systems-level research that provides the foundation for his development of recovery system standard dimensions. The author delineates the essential services in recovery-oriented systems of care, including treatment, crisis intervention, case management, rehabilitation, rights protection, basic support, self-help, and wellness/prevention.[47] The standards incorporate the importance of recovery as the basis of the system and provide guidance and direction to reinforce the development of recovery-oriented systems of care. The standards are grouped by systems-level dimensions (for specific detail on the essential services and standards, please see Anthony, 2000):[48]

- Design
- Evaluation
- Leadership
- Management
- Integration
- Comprehensiveness
- Consumer involvement
- Cultural relevance
- Advocacy
- Training
- Funding
- Access

Jacobson and Curtis (2000) reviewed existing literature on the conceptualizations of recovery that are integrated within recovery-oriented systems of care for the mental health field:[49]

- Recovery is generally seen as a process. It does not represent a cure, but a state of being and becoming.
- The path to recovery is highly singular or unique; no two people will have identical paths or use the same benchmarks to measure their journeys.
- In contrast to the passivity of being a patient or a voiceless recipient of services, recovery is active and requires that an individual take personal responsibility for his or her own recovery, often in collaboration with friends, family, supporters, and professionals.
- A recovery orientation includes an emphasis on choice, a concept that encompasses support for autonomous action, the requirement that the individual have a range of opportunities from which to choose and full information about those choices, and increasing personal responsibility for the consequences of choice.
- The emotional essence of recovery is hope, a promise that things can and do change, that today is not the way it will always be.
- A key theme is that of meaning, or the discovery of purpose and direction in one's life. The search for meaning is highly personal. For some people meaning may be reflected through work or social relationships. Others derive meaning from advocacy and political action. For others, the pursuit of meaning takes on strongly spiritual elements.

Finally, as discussed by Barton (1998), the three models for delivering care within a fragmented mental health system—the medical, rehabilitation, and community support system models—are responsible for the outcomes of care.[50] The recovery philosophy articulates the "process through which this occurs in partnership with the recovering consumer. From this perspective, the consumer-centered recovery philosophy is the umbrella over all models, disciplines, practices, and activities in the hospital and the community."[51] In this philosophy, system principles include:

- Empowerment of staff and consumers,
- Integration of the rehabilitation and medical model services across hospital and community settings,
- Provision of client-centered services,
- Validation of client choice,
- Generation of hope, and
- Collaboration and partnership, e.g., consumers, professionals, and disciplines.

5. RESEARCH SUPPORTING THE PRINCIPLES OF RECOVERY AND SYSTEMS OF CARE ELEMENTS

Previous research efforts have outlined principles of effective addictions treatment. In 1999, the National Institute on Drug Abuse (NIDA) produced a research-based guide entitled *Principles of Drug Addiction Treatment*. It identified 13 principles that research has found to be associated with effective addictions treatment:[52]

1. No single treatment is appropriate for all individuals.
2. Treatment needs to be readily available.
3. Effective treatment attends to multiple needs of the individual, not just his or her drug use.
4. An individual's treatment and services plan must be assessed continually and modified as necessary to ensure that the plan meets the person's changing needs.
5. Remaining in treatment for an adequate period of time is critical for treatment effectiveness.
6. Counseling (individual and/or group) and other behavioral therapies are critical components of effective treatment for addiction.
7. Medications are an important element of treatment for many patients, especially when combined with counseling and other behavioral therapies.
8. Addicted or drug-abusing individuals with coexisting mental disorders should have both disorders treated in an integrated way.
9. Medical detoxification is only the first stage of addictions treatment and by itself does little to change long-term drug use.
10. Treatment does not need to be voluntary to be effective.
11. Possible drug use during treatment must be monitored continuously.
12. Treatment programs should provide assessment for HIV/AIDS, hepatitis B and C, tuberculosis, and other infectious diseases, and counseling to help patients modify or change behaviors that place themselves or others at the risk of infection.
13. Recovery from drug addiction can be a long-term process and frequently requires multiple episodes of treatment.

NIDA's principles focus on the process of delivering effective treatment. The National Summit on Recovery's 12 principles of recovery provides guidelines on the process of and outcomes associated with recovery. The NIDA principles relate most closely to the following principles of recovery:

- **There are many pathways to recovery.** The pathway to recovery may include one or more episodes of psychosocial and/or pharmacological treatment. For some, recovery involves neither treatment nor involvement with mutual aid groups. Recovery is a process of change that permits an individual to make healthy choices and improve the quality of his or her life.
- **Recovery is holistic.** Recovery is a process through which one gradually achieves greater balance of mind, body, and spirit in relation to other aspects of one's life, including family, work, and community.
- **Recovery exists on a continuum of improved health and wellness.** Recovery is not a linear process. It is based on continual growth and improved functioning.
- **Recovery involves a process of healing and self-redefinition.** Recovery is a holistic healing process in which one develops a positive and meaningful sense of identity.
- **Recovery is a reality.** It can, will, and does happen.

6. Research Supporting the Principles of Recovery

> **There are many pathways to recovery.**
> Individuals are unique with specific needs, strengths, goals, health attitudes, behaviors and expectations for recovery. Pathways to recovery are highly personal, and generally involve a redefinition of identity in the face of crisis or a process of progressive change. Furthermore, pathways are often social, grounded in cultural beliefs or traditions and involve informal community resources, which provide support for sobriety. The pathway to recovery may include one or more episodes of psychosocial and/or pharmacological treatment.
>
> For some, recovery involves neither treatment nor involvement with mutual aid groups. Recovery is a process of change that permits an individual to make healthy choices and improve the quality of his or her life.

Research has shown that there are a variety of methods that assist individuals in their process of recovery.[53,54] Some people recover naturally; others recover through treatment and/or the assistance of self-help and mutual aid groups.[55]

Natural recovery involves using one's own personal resources to resolve one's addictions without the use of treatment or involvement in a mutual aid or self-help group. It is believed to be the most common recovery pathway.[56-64]

In studies examining the existence and success of natural recovery, alcohol was the most studied substance, with heroin a distant second.[65] Research has shown that natural recovery is a viable and successful pathway for people with shorter and less severe substance use problems and disorders and for those with higher incomes and more stable social and occupational supports and resources.[66-72] Additionally, individuals who recover naturally typically have fewer interpersonal conflicts and rely less on avoidance coping.[73-75]

Granfield and Cloud (2001) attribute the success of natural recovery to an individual's social capital, which they define as "the benefits that accrue to an individual as a result of the network of personal contacts and associations that surround them."[76, p.1566] The "natural communities of friends, family members, and relatives, and the social capital available through these connections, contribute significantly" to recovery success.[77]

Longitudinal studies have repeatedly shown that substance use problems and disorders treatment is associated with major reductions in substance use, problems, and costs to society, and improved patient recovery.[78-85] Of individuals with chronic dependence who achieved sustained recovery, the majority did so after participating in treatment— cannabis (43 percent), cocaine (61 percent), alcohol (81 percent), and heroin (92 percent).[86,87] For some, treatment is part of the recovery process, while for others, they recover outside of the treatment system without the aid of treatment.

Participation in mutual aid groups has also been shown to be effective in supporting recovery.[88-98] Laudet, Savage, and Mahmood (2002) and Scott, Dennis, and Foss (2005) found that for many individuals in long-term recovery, recovery coaches, 12-step programs, spirituality, and social and community support are integral to sustaining recovery.[99, 100] One of the most widely studied self-help/12-step groups is Alcoholics Anonymous (AA). Research has shown that patients who attend AA regularly experience better short-term alcohol-related outcomes than do patients who attend infrequently or irregularly.[101-103] Furthermore, ongoing participation in AA contributes to continued improvement of substance use disorder symptoms.[104-106]

Methadone is one of the most thoroughly studied pharmaceuticals in modern medicine. Methadone maintenance therapy (MMT) is one of the most widespread treatment approaches, with 179,000 individuals enrolled in MMT (out of an estimated 900,000 opiate-dependent persons in the United States) and 100,000 individuals receiving another form of treatment.[107] Methadone, combined with psychosocial support, leads to improved outcomes, such as decreased death rates, reduced transmission of sexually transmitted diseases, eliminated or reduced illicit opiate use, reduced criminal activity, enhanced productive behavior through employment and academic/vocational functioning, and improved global health and social functioning.[108]

> **Recovery is self-directed and empowering.**
> While the pathway to recovery may involve one or more periods of time when activities are directed or guided to a substantial degree by others, recovery is fundamentally a self-directed process. The person in recovery is the "agent of recovery" and has the authority to exercise choices and make decisions based on his or her recovery goals that have an impact on the process. The process of recovery leads individuals toward the highest level of autonomy of which they are capable. Through self-empowerment, individuals become optimistic about life goals.

Doty, Kasper, and Litvak (1996) and Tilly and Wiener (2001a, 2001b), reporting on the results of initiatives in several States (California, Colorado, Kansas, Maine, Michigan, Oregon, Washington, and Wisconsin), demonstrated the effectiveness of consumer-directed services.[109-111] These evaluations show that clients who direct their own care express greater satisfaction over the services they choose. Moreover, participants in these State consumer-directed programs perceived that quality of care either improved as a result of consumer direction or at least did not suffer. An evaluation of an Arkansas consumer-directed care program found that individuals in the program were less likely than control subjects to have unmet needs, were at least as safe from adverse events and health problems, and were more likely to be satisfied with life.[112]

Research shows that a sense of self-efficacy is critical to successful self-management, where individuals direct and manage their own care of a variety of chronic illnesses. This is also the case in achieving improvements in health outcomes,[113-116] and self-management has been shown to be an important component of recovery from substance use.[117]

Morgenstern, Labouvie, McCrady, Kahler, and Frey (1997) found that maintaining motivation and self-efficacy for abstinence and increasing active coping post treatment were predictive of more favorable outcomes.[118] Motivational interviewing (MI) has been shown to decrease substance use and improve outcomes.[119] MI is based on a partnership between the provider and the individual receiving services, and it acknowledges that individual's personal responsibility and freedom of choice.[120] It replaces the concept of "resistance" with that of "ambivalence." MI allows individuals to explore their own goals and take an active role in treatment,[121,122] thereby assisting individuals in changing their substance use behavior.[123] The clinician using MI assists the individual in clarifying personal goals, identifying discrepancies between the individual's current reality and his or her goals, and developing strategies to achieve those goals.[124, 125]

> **Recovery involves a personal recognition of the need for change and transformation.**
>
> Individuals must accept that a problem exists and be willing to take steps to address it; these steps usually involve seeking help for a substance use disorder. The process of change can involve physical, emotional, intellectual and spiritual aspects of the person's life.

Research shows that the motivation to change drug-using behavior is a major contributing factor to a successful recovery process,[126-130] and the effect of motivation varies based on severity of an individual's substance use disorderJoe, Simpson, and Broome (1999) identified motivation as the best predictor of engagement and retention.[132] The substance-using individual must accept that he or she has a problem, make a conscious choice to change, and be willing and motivated to take action to change his or her behavior.[133]

> **Recovery is holistic.**
>
> Recovery is a process through which one gradually achieves greater balance of mind, body and spirit in relation to other aspects of one's life, including family, work and community.

Some literature demonstrates that the integration of the physical, emotional, and spiritual realms of an individual is influential in the quest for recovery.[134] Alternative (e.g., acupuncture) and traditional medicine approaches for substance use treatment and recovery programs promote a balance between mind, body, and spirit, and other aspects of an individual's life, and have been shown to be valuable in helping an individual achieve recovery.[135] For example, individuals who participated in a comprehensive, holistic, therapeutic community that offered many specialized services had sustained positive outcomes, including abstinence from drug and alcohol use 12 months post treatment.[136]

> **Recovery has cultural dimensions.**
>
> Each person's recovery process is unique and impacted by cultural beliefs and traditions. A person's cultural experience often shapes the recovery path that is right for him or her.

The literature demonstrates that an individual's culture plays a vital role in his/her life and health status and that culture must be acknowledged, addressed, and effectively utilized in recovery. [137-141] Cross-cultural studies have demonstrated the importance of delivering culturally competent care. [142,143] Research shows that culturally competent care improves recovery and remission rates for minority populations who are at risk for relapse. [144-146]

Flores (2000), in his meta-analysis of research on implications of culture on clinical care, concludes that culture has significant implications on the patient-provider relationship and the delivery of efficacious care. [147] He further states that it is essential for providers to consider a patient's culture and linguistic issues; the failure to do so has been shown to result in inefficiencies and inequalities in patient care, such as "inaccurate histories, decreased satisfaction with care, nonadherence, poor continuity of care, less preventive screening, miscommunication," [148] which leads to repercussions in care delivery.

Traditional theories of counseling and treatment are reflective of the Western cultures. It is essential that providers develop awareness, knowledge, and skills appropriate to the client's culture. [149,150] This is particularly important when the counselor is working with individuals who do not share the counselor's racial or ethnic heritage. [151,152] Some scholars have argued that other aspects of culture, including sexual orientation, ethnicity, religion, and heritage, are also important. [153,154] Researchers believe that recovery African-American Asians are lower than other populations due to the failure of treatment providers and researchers a physical phenomenon. [155-157]

> **Recovery exists on a continuum of improved health and wellness.**
> Recovery is not a linear process. It is based on continual growth and improved functioning. It may involve relapse and other setbacks, which are a natural part of the continuum but not inevitable outcomes. Wellness is the result of improved care and balance of mind, body and spirit. It is a product of the recovery process.

The literature consistently demonstrates that for many people, substance use problems and disorders are chronic conditions involving cycles of relapse and treatment readmissions over multiple years.[158-163] Scholars and researchers agree that recovery is a developmental and continuous process that varies from person to person.[164, 165] Individuals continuously grow and improve their functioning throughout the recovery process. Additionally, individuals benefit from lessons learned throughout the process.[166]

> **Recovery emerges from hope and gratitude.**
> Individuals in or seeking recovery often gain hope from those who share their search for or experience of recovery. They see that people can and do overcome the obstacles that confront them and they cultivate gratitude for the opportunities that each day of recovery offers.

Several authors have written about growth beyond maintaining abstinence or management of the problem, often describing theoretical frameworks and specific practices and techniques that help management of the problem and promote wider growth.[167-175] Irving, Seidner, Burling, Pagliarini, and Robbins-Sisco (1998) found that greater hope and increased goal-oriented thinking were positively correlated to length of time abstinent, quality of life, and self-efficacy.[176] Additionally, listening to peers share experiences about how they dealt successfully with drug-related problems gave individuals in recovery confidence in dealing with their own situations.[177]

In a qualitative study, Hewitt (2004) describes the posttraumatic growth that individuals experience after discontinuing alcohol and drug use.[178] His study expands a phenomenon reflected in the AA concept of gratitude:[179] recovering alcoholics often report viewing their alcoholism as a gift that brought them to a greater sense of wholeness, fulfillment, or self-actualization than they feel they would have achieved without having to confront the addiction. In his study, Hewitt found that many individuals marked a contrast between the "craziness" of their previous lives, which were devoted to drugs or alcohol, and the calmness, stability, and sanity that were more characteristic of their current post addiction lives.[180]

The importance of having hope and believing in the possibility of a renewed sense of self and purpose is an essential component of recovery;[181-187] this hope must be accompanied by a desire and motivation to recover.[188,189] Young and Ensing (1999) found that seeking out a source of hope and inspiration helps individuals desire change and foster motivation to embark on and/or sustain a process of change.[190]

> **Recovery involves a process of healing and self-redefinition.**
> Recovery is a holistic healing process in which one develops a positive and meaningful sense of identity.

McMillen, Howard, Nower, and Chung (2001) identified positive by-products of the struggle with substance use problems and disorders, including changes in life priorities and increases in self-efficacy, family closeness, closeness with others, spirituality, and compassion.[191] Many consumers view recovery as a process of discovering and fostering self-empowerment, learning self-redefinition, returning to basic functioning, and improving quality of life.[192]

> **Recovery involves addressing discrimination and transcending shame and stigma.**
> Recovery is a process by which people confront and strive to overcome stigma.

Stigma and discrimination have implications for an individual's ability to receive care and continue on the path of recovery.[193] Based on combined data from SAMHSA's 2004 and 2005 National Survey on Drug Use and Health (NSDUH), stigma was cited as the reason for not accessing treatment by 18.5 percent of persons who needed and sought treatment but did not receive it.[194]

Clinical practices may not be the most efficient way to reduce stigma, which is a major barrier to care, because the causes of stigma exist both within and outside of the health care system.[195-197] Furthermore, societal stigma is viewed as one of the major barriers to recovery.[198]

While stigma is seen as a major barrier to accessing treatment, it also plays a role in affecting outcomes of treatment and access to services for individuals in recovery.[199 -201] Link, Struening, Neese-Todd, Asmussen, and Phelan (2001) found that the stigma associated with mental illness puts people more at risk for low self-esteem.[202] According to the *Christian Science Monitor*, experts in treatment and recovery estimate that when recovering individuals are honest about their drug histories, they will be turned down for a job 75 percent of the time.[203] Additionally, a California survey found that 59 percent of employers surveyed said they would never hire anyone with a felony conviction.[204]

Recovery is supported by peers and allies.

A common denominator in the recovery process is the presence and involvement of people who contribute hope and support and suggest strategies and resources for change. Peers, as well as family members and other allies, form vital support networks for people in recovery. Providing service to others and experiencing mutual healing help create a community of support among those in recovery.

Evaluation data and research studies point to the benefits of peer-based recovery support services for consumers, individuals who provide the services, and the delivery system.[205-213] An individual's sustained recovery is often influenced by his or her social interactions.[214] Peers have been shown to be integral in facilitating abstinence and preventing relapse for individuals with substance use conditions.[215-220] Jason, Davis, Ferrari, and Bishop (2001) and Humphreys, Huebsch, Finney, and Moos (1999) found that processes of social support mediate the transition from recovery initiation to lifelong recovery maintenance;[221,222] furthermore, research shows that poor social supports detrimentally impact recovery and place individuals at risk for relapse.[223, 224]

Mutual aid (or "self-help") groups have been shown to play a significant role in the process of recovery.[225-236] These peer-based support groups require no admission process or specified length of participation and are less formalized than other types of peer recovery services. The probability of stable remission rates has been shown to rise in concert with the number of recovery mutual aid groups attended in the first 3 years of recovery.[237] Additionally, active and continued participation in self-help groups has been shown to improve recovery outcomes.[238-246]

A longitudinal study of Oxford House recovery homes suggests that receiving abstinence support, guidance, and information from recovery home members committed to the goal of long-term sobriety enhances residents' abstinence and reduces the residents' probability of relapse.[247, 248]

Recovery involves (re)joining and (re)building a life in the community.

Recovery involves a process of building or rebuilding what a person has lost or never had due to his or her condition and its consequences.

Recovery involves creating a life within the limitation imposed by that condition. Recovery is building or rebuilding healthy family, social and personal relationships. Those in recovery often achieve improvements in the quality of their life, such as obtaining education, employment and housing. They also increasingly become involved in constructive roles in the community through helping others, productive acts and other contributions.

The basic element in the process of recovery is the reclaiming of one's life in the community and the realization that one's self needs to be restored with a reawakening of old identities and establishment of new ones.[249] Individuals entering recovery must often work to reintegrate themselves with their families and communities,[250] while disengaging themselves from relationships, activities, and settings associated with their addictive behavior. By detaching oneself from the previous environment, an individual can find a satisfying job, non-substance-using friends, and networks of people who may be in recovery.[251-253] Personal resources,[254] positive influences of family,[255] and social and community support[256] have been shown to be critical factors in establishing and maintaining recovery. Granfield and Cloud (2001) posited that recovery capital, which are defined as resources that support people's recovery from substance use problems and disorders, and the inclusion of a strong social network of sober friends and family members, employment, education and a range of coping skills, improves an individual's capacity to successfully recover.[257,258]

Interventions that restructure the patient's life in the community, such as parole, methadone maintenance, and self-help groups, have also been associated with sustained abstinence.[259] As a part of one's recovery process and to incorporate oneself into an environment that supports their recovery, many individuals make fundamental changes to their personal, professional, and social network environments.[260-264]

> **Recovery is a reality.**
> It can, will, and does happen.

Many agree that recovery is a continuous, lifelong process.[265-267] Epidemiologic studies show that, on average, 58 percent of individuals with chronic substance dependence achieve sustained recovery.[268-271] Recovery rates for individuals with substance use problems and disorders differ by study and vary widely, from 30 percent,[272] 41 percent,[273] 48 percent,[274] 59 percent,[275] 63 percent,[276] to 72 percent.[277]

A national survey conducted on behalf of Faces and Voices of Recovery found that approximately half of individuals who self-identified as "in recovery" or "formally addicted to" alcohol and other drugs reported being in recovery more than 5 years, and 34 percent reported 10 years or more of stable recovery.[278]

7. Research Supporting the Systems of Care Elements

> **Person-centered**
> Recovery-oriented systems of care will be person-centered. Individuals will have a menu of stage-appropriate choices that fit their needs throughout the recovery process. Choices can include spiritual supports that fit with the individual's recovery needs.

A number of studies have shown that people become more committed to a course of treatment if they are allowed to choose between several alternatives rather than are forced to select a given option.[279] Patient choice of care is important to the individual patient and improves engagement with treatment and continuing care services.[280] Several studies have indicated that clients who were given a choice of treatment options showed greater acceptance of treatment and higher rates of recovery at follow-up.[281-286]

Researchers have reported that clients who had a choice of treatment had improved treatment processes and post treatment outcomes. Individuals who were provided with the option to choose their treatment services were more likely to work harder in treatment,[287] have more contact with their treatment program,[288] and better adhere to program requirements than individuals who were not given a choice of treatment.[289] Those who had treatment options were also less likely to drop out of treatment.[290]

Inclusive of family and other ally involvement

Recovery-oriented systems of care will acknowledge the important role that families and other allies can play. Family and other allies will be incorporated, when appropriate, in the recovery planning and support process. They can constitute a source of support to assist individuals in entering and maintaining recovery. Additionally, systems need to address the treatment, recovery and other support needs of families and other allies.

Research has demonstrated that involvement of concerned others can lead to improved outcomes in both alcohol[291-293] and drug[294] treatment. These connections may enhance individual's self-efficacy and reduce the probability of relapse.[295] In a review by McCrady (2004), it was shown that family and ally involvement in treatment was associated with more positive treatment outcomes in a variety of alcohol-dependent populations.[296]

Family and ally support and healthy and productive relationships nurture long-term recovery.[297] The family has been shown to be a key determinant of an individual's commitment and ability to achieve recovery.[298] An individual's family and other allies can be active participants, sources of strength, and resources in recovery and can provide a central role in maintenance of recovery.[299-304]

The level of social support that an individual receives has been directly associated with engagement indicators and treatment completion.[305] Finney, Noyes, Coutts, and Moos (1998) found that recovery-oriented support may foster greater self-efficacy and longer abstinence.[306] The positive consequences linked to these associations may be the result of individuals acquiring effective coping strategies and greater support from other recovering individuals.[307-309] Furthermore, it has been shown that social support, particularly through interactions with individuals in similar situations, produces positive health implications.[310]

In a randomized controlled trial, it was shown that spouse involvement, regardless of the type and intensity of therapy utilized, was an effective intervention for enhancing compliance to disulfiram,[311] reducing total alcohol consumption[312-314] and maintaining treatment gains following discharge.[315] Higgins, Budney, Bickel, and Badger (1994) found that cocaine-abusing individuals participating in community reinforcement with a significant other had better outcomes than those who chose not to bring a significant other.[316]

Individualized and comprehensive services across the lifespan

Recovery-oriented systems of care will be individualized, comprehensive, stage-appropriate, and flexible. Systems will adapt to the needs of individuals, rather than requiring individuals to adapt to them. They will be designed to support recovery across the lifespan. The approach to substance use disorders will change from an acute-based model to one that manages chronic disorders over a lifetime.

Research has shown that access to and receipt of a comprehensive array of medical, psychological, and social services improves engagement, retention, and treatment outcomes.[317-320] For example, access to housing, employment, and legal systems has positively aided in the treatment of substance use problems and sustained abstinence.[321-323]

Studies find that when an individual's full array of needs (e.g., food, clothing, housing, transportation, medical care, childcare, and family, psychiatric, educational, and vocational concerns) are met, short-and long-term outcomes, including retention in treatment and reduction in substance use, are improved.[324-326] Additionally, if individuals' distinct needs are addressed, outcomes are improved.[327-330]

Similarly, individuals presenting to substance use problems and disorders treatment with comorbid psychiatric or medical conditions often have great difficulty sustaining recovery unless these conditions are fully assessed and addressed during treatment and continuing care.[331, 332]

Recovery across the Lifespan

Due to inherent differences, issues of gender, race, and age should be considered in the treatment and recovery process.[333-336] As individuals age, their health needs and social relationships evolve and their cognitive processes change.[337, 338] Treatment approaches and social support mechanisms need to be developmentally appropriate, taking into account the age of individuals.[339] Adolescent, adult, and elderly substance users differ in many ways and have unique issues and concerns that must be addressed through specific treatment and recovery planning.[340-344] At different stages in life, an individual's drug and alcohol use often stems from different causes and requires age-appropriate treatments.[345-350] Because of their unique developmental issues, adolescent, adult, and elderly users must be treated differently, with the variation taken into account in their treatment and recovery plans. Moreover, treatment approaches should address the nuances of each individual's experience, and their cognitive, emotional, physical, social, and moral development.[351,352]

Research shows that the types of substances that individuals misuse varies with age. Older adults, for example, more often misuse alcohol and prescription and over-the-counter drugs, while younger substance abusers more often use illicit drugs.[353-355] Adolescents are vulnerable due to their developmental stage, but multiple biological, psychological, and social changes associated with the aging process also make the elderly uniquely vulnerable to substance abuse problems.[356-359]

Natural recovery is most often seen in individuals with patterns of substance use that are moderate to mild or of short duration and is most often encountered among two age cohorts: 1) young adults whose use discontinues or is substantially reduced with maturation and assumption of adult role responsibilities, and 2) later-life adults who change behavior in response to the cumulative consequences of substance use.[360,361] (See also the discussion of natural recovery in Section 6.)

> **Systems anchored in the community**
> Recovery-oriented systems of care will be nested in the community for the purpose of enhancing the availability and support capacities of families, intimate social networks, community-based institutions and other people in recovery.

Research shows that social and community resources promote better recovery outcomes.[362] Healthy and productive environments are nurturing of recovery,[363,364] and the presence of strong social networks during and after treatment consistently to sustained reductions in substance use-367] Strong social networks are particularly important as a counterbalance to the social pressures within high-drug-using networks and neighborhoods.[368-371]

To improve individuals communities resources social support-374] Comprehensive, easily accessible recovery support service programs located in high-need communities with staff functioning in multiple roles using culturally competent interventions have been shown to improve recovery outcomes for individuals with children.[375] Employment and stable housing have been found to improve self-esteem and support reintegration into mainstream society and thereby to support recovery.[376-381]

Community-based care systems provide opportunities for transitions between levels and types of care in a cost-effective manner and improve long-term health outcomes.[382,383] The Team for the Assessment of Psychiatric Services (TAPS) examined the health outcomes and quality of care for individuals discharged into the community psychiatric hospitalizations.[384] Of 523 individuals still alive at the 5-year follow-up, 90 percent were still living in the community, and few individuals reported criminal justice system involvement or homelessness.[385]

Harrison (2001) and Knight, Simpson, and Hiller (1999) found that, among offenders reentering the community, participation in an in-prison treatment and in a post release, community-based aftercare program was associated with positive outcomes.[386, 387]

Continuity of care

Recovery-oriented systems of care will offer a continuum of care, including pretreatment, treatment, continuing care and support throughout recovery. Individuals will have a full range of stage-appropriate services from which to choose at any point in the recovery process.

Continuity of care is particularly important in treating chronic and complex diseases where several providers may be involved in the provision of care.[388] Continuity of care is characterized by care from one doctor or team, coordinated through a common purpose and plan.[389] Furthermore, continuity of care is significantly related to positive treatment outcomes,[390] since continued attachment to treatment is consistently related to better outcomes.[391]

Continuing care includes services accessed post discharge from treatment lower intensity. It provides sustained access treatment and recoverypromotes continued abstinence and recovery. Empirical research has demonstrated that continuing care contributes to improved treatment outcomes.[392,393] Gruber, Fleetwood, and Herring (2001) highlighted the efficacy and the positive effects of a continuing care program designed to assist the substance-affected family.[394] Continuing care has been shown to be effective in assisting individuals in starting and maintaining recovery.[395] The utilization of continuing care improves long-term recovery outcomes;[396,397] without continuing care, individuals are more likely to relapse.[398,399]

Linkage and retention in continuing care have been shown to improve long-term abstinence from a variety of substances.[400] Studies have shown that onsite medical consultation, team-based approaches, and facilitated referrals to primary care independently have a substantial positive impact on linkage to medical care and its quality for persons with mental and addictive disorders.[401, 402] For example, participation in community services has been associated with engagement in outpatient treatment and better treatment outcomes.[403-413] Individuals who become more engaged in outpatient care in the community and self-help groups tend to experience better short-term abstinence outcomes.[414]

Transitional services are particularly important for correctional populations.[415, 416] Substance use disorder treatment, when provided in conjunction with credible sanctions against drug offenses, job training and placement, and advocacy services, has been shown to decrease recidivism rates and improve reentry from correctional institutions into the community for recovering drug offenders.[417] Completion of aftercare services by offenders has been shown to improve recovery outcomes.[418-420]

Partnership-consultant relationships

Recovery-oriented systems of care will be patterned after a partnership-consultant model that focuses more on collaboration and less on hierarchy. Systems will be designed so that individuals feel empowered to direct their own recovery.

Research shows that supportive therapeutic and trusting relationships enhance engagement and retention.[421-424] Early therapeutic alliances appear to be a consistent predictor of engagement and retention in treatment.[425] Providers must convey hope in their interactions with clients and develop individualized treatment or recovery plans that incorporate clients' goals and are designed to support increased patient/client autonomy.[426]

A partnership-consultant relationship is utilized to encourage patient self-managementPatient self-management requires the clinician to utilize a "collaborative care model of practice in which the patient and clinician are equal partners, with equal expertise."[428] In the collaborative care model, the clinician brings medical expertise and "patients are experts in their own lives and in what concerns them and motivates and enables them to make changes in their lives,"[429] thereby creating a therapeutic alliance with patients as their principal caregivers.

A therapeutic alliance between providers and patients embraces a more empathetic approach where providers enhance their clients' involvement in service delivery and recovery.[430] Success of counseling is related to the quality of a working alliance and utilization of a patient-centered focus with therapist empathy, warmth, and genuineness.[431] A positive working alliance, reported by either the client or therapist, is a significant predictor of treatment participation and substance use behavior post treatment.[432,433] The association of a therapeutic relationship with positive outcomes is consistently reported, and there is a positive relationship between therapeutic alliances and outcomes. Moreover, "counselors who are confrontational or use confrontational interventions consistently" have worse outcomes.[434]

Studies confirming this have been performed across settings (residential, outpatient continuing care, and office based) and approaches (medication and family treatment-439] Ilgen, Tiet, Finney, and Moos (2006) and Ilgen, McKellar, Moos, and Finney (2006) found that a positive therapeutic alliance counteracted the negative impact of low baseline self-efficacy and low motivation in some people.[440,441] Carten (1996) observed that the development of positive relationship designed service contracts, shared planning, staff encouragement, nonjudgmental attitudes, and nonpunitive responses to relapse, improved success for mothers in recovery.[442]

Strength-based

Recovery-oriented systems of care will emphasize individual strengths, assets and resiliencies.

The strengths perspective emphasizes building on the client's assets, desires, abilities, and resources to assist the client in the recovery process.[443] Additionally, the strengths perspective demonstrates the importance and respect for the client's way of thinking and dealing with life situations. This perspective assumes that each individual has the capacity to draw from a variety of resources, skills, and motivations to focus on their strengths and create change in their lives.[444-447] Through examining the efficacy of combining intensive strengths-based case management services with an established program, Siegal and colleagues found that individuals who received strengths-based case management services had improved retention in treatment, lower reported drug and alcohol use, and better outcomes related to criminality and employment than those who did not receive the intervention.[448-450]

Culturally responsive

Recovery-oriented systems of care will be culturally sensitive, competent and responsive. There will be recognition that beliefs and customs are diverse and can impact the outcomes of recovery efforts. In addition, the cultures of those who support the recovering individual affect the recovery process.

Professional ethical guidelines and recently developed multicultural competencies for working with diverse populations suggest that the delivery of culturally competent services is integral to the delivery of quality and effective services.[451] Cultural competence has become a very important focus in the health services delivery field, as demonstrated by the U.S. Department of Health and Human Services, Office of Minority Health's standards project on Culturally and Linguistically Appropriate Services (CLAS).[452]

Ignoring culture can result in many negative consequences, including missed opportunities for screening, difficulties resulting from differing responses to medication, lack of clinician knowledge about alternative and traditional remedies, diagnostic errors resulting from miscommunication, and disruptions in services.[453-457] Minority Americans have different health experiences than nonminorities.[458] Moreover, nonminority Americans have different experiences from each other in the health care setting, even when they have similar medical conditions and insurance coverage.[459-466]

Gender-and culture-based approaches provide more effective substance abuse treatment for all individuals with substance use problems and disorders, particularly for African-Americans, Hispanics, and Asians and their families.[467-469] Longshore, Grills, and Annon (1999) found that individuals in a more culturally congruent intervention were more involved in counseling sessions, more willing to self-disclose, more motivated to seek help for drug use–associated problems, and more prepared for change.[470] Campbell and Alexander (2002) found that individuals treated in culturally competent substance abuse treatment practices had higher rates of specific medical and psychosocial services, such as medical exams and financial services, but they concluded that the practices may not be uniformly effective in promoting utilization of all services.[471] Gender-and culture-specific care needs in relation to social structure, ethno-history, and cultural context have been shown to influence women's health and well-being as they move through recovery.[472]

Responsiveness to personal belief systems

Recovery-oriented systems of care will respect the spiritual, religious and/or secular beliefs of those they serve and provide linkages to an array of recovery options that are consistent with these beliefs.

Many researchers have documented the value of individuals' spiritual, religious, and secular beliefs in supporting recovery.[473-481] Religious involvement and spiritual (re)engagement appear to be correlated with and facilitate the process of recovery.[482-484]

Spirituality and faith, through their associations with cognitive processes, create more positive health outcomes, including optimistic life orientation, higher resilience to stress, lower levels of anxiety, and positive effective coping skills.[485] Evidence shows that spirituality and faith may facilitate the process of recovery[486-488] and promote improvements in long-term recovery.[489] Spirituality, religiousness, and life meaning "enhance coping, confer hope for the future, and provide a heightened sense of control, security, and stability; they offer support and strength to resist the opportunity to use substances, all of which are very much needed to initiate and maintain recovery."[490,p.15] Furthermore, many individuals in recovery cite strength acquired from religion and spirituality as main factors in contributing to their long-term recovery,[491, 492] as a source of personal strength, and as a self-protection mechanism.[493]

Commitment to peer recovery support services

Recovery-oriented systems of care will include peer recovery support services. Individuals with personal experience of recovery will provide these valuable services.

Research on peer support / mutual support groups / recovering consumers as providers of alcohol and drug treatment services shows that the use of peer support is effective in helping individuals through recovery.[494-496] Evidence shows that seeing or visualizing those similar to oneself performing activities typically increases one's belief in one's own ability to perform those activities[497] and facilitates successful management of one's chronic illness.[498] Moreover, peer support has been identified in the Chronic Care Model as a method to support patients in their illness self-management.[499,500] Peer recovery support services "foster recovery in a relational, mutually-enhancing, and safe context."[501, p.171]

Involvement in mutual aid groups provides an opportunity for individuals to participate in drug-and alcohol-free activities as role models to others, rewards their own abstinence, and helps enhance individuals' personal and social resources.[502-504] Twelve-step involvement has been related to positive outcomes, including decreased substance use,[505-511] enhanced psychosocial adjustment,[512-514] and lower health care costs.[515] Moreover, 12-step participation as a continuing care activity has been shown to be effective for long-term abstinence.[516-519] Self-help groups help sustain recovery[520-523] and provide a community that strives to be drug-free with a structured mechanism for continuous abstinence or recovery.[524]

AA affiliation has been associated with self-efficacy and positive coping, which has been linked to better outcomes.[525, 526] Rational Recovery, a self-help approach started by a clinical social worker in 1986, is intended for persons with all types of addictive disorders. It adopts cognitive approaches and has been shown to be successful in engaging substance users and promoting abstinence among members.[527]

For some dual diagnosis patients, 12-step interventions have been found to be more effective in decreasing alcohol use and increasing social interactions than self-management.[528] (For further information on self-management, please see discussion on page 16.)

Inclusion of the voices and experiences of recovering individuals and their families

The voices and experiences of people in recovery and their family members will contribute to the design and implementation of recovery-oriented systems of care. People in recovery and their family members will be included among decision-makers and have oversight responsibilities for service provision. Recovering individuals and family members will be prominently and authentically represented on advisory councils, boards, task forces and committees at the Federal, State and local levels.

Community involvement with public health planning and implementation has been shown to be integral to improving community health.[529, 530] Additionally, with regard to improving public safety, the voices of consumers have played a large role in restructuring medical systems to better promote consumer, provider, and system safety.[531] In these movements worldwide, consumers have played key roles in defining the priorities, providing personal expertise, and reforming patient safety criteria of health care systems.[532] The patient safety movement is an excellent example of how partnerships among consumers and providers of care were instrumental in improving operational and systemic deficiencies.[533]

The rationale for seeking participation by consumers falls into three categories: 1) to improve services and decisions, 2) to gain legitimization and/or community compliance, and 3) to bring about social change with the redistribution of power or resources.[534] Furthermore, individuals with a "particular disease become more aggressive in voicing their desire not only for more response from government and the health care system, but also for more influence over policy decisions at the macro level and treatment decisions at the micro level…[for example,] by people with disabilities and their families and those initially affected by human immunodeficiency virus/acquired immunodeficiency syndrome (HIV/AIDS)."[535, p.216] Research shows that giving mental health consumers a significant role in shaping services, policies, and research improves services.[536]

Some government agencies have mandated the involvement of affected populations in policy decisions through advisory groups and planning councils.[537] Little systematic research as to the effectiveness of the involvement of consumers on decision-making has been conducted.[538]

Integrated services

Recovery-oriented systems of care will coordinate and/or integrate efforts across service systems to achieve an integrated process that responds effectively to the individual's unique constellation of strengths, desires and needs.

Integrating care has been shown to optimize recovery outcomes and improve the cost-effectiveness of delivering services.[539-541] Collaboration between and integration across services systems and agencies has improved the probability of individual and family recovery.[542] Research has demonstrated the efficacy and effectiveness of providing onsite primary medical care and ancillary services in the addictions treatment setting[543-545] and integrating addictions services into other settings.[546,547]

Patients in an enhanced program that used case managers who coordinated and expedited the use of medical screening, housing assistance, parenting classes, and employment services had significantly fewer physical and mental health problems, better social functioning, and less substance use at 6 months after treatment than did individuals who were not in the enhanced program.[548,549]

Programs that are more effective with dually diagnosed individuals tend to have a combined treatment orientation; adopt a more tolerant and persuasive, rather than confrontational stance; use peer modeling in group psychotherapy; and provide continuity of care through assertive case management and after-care.[550-552] Additionally, individuals with co-occurring substance use problems and disorders and medical conditions have been shown to benefit from an integrated medical and substance abuse treatment program, with increased rates of abstinence, compared with individuals without co-occurring medical problems.[553,554]

Families and children at risk often present with a complex array of needs that require the provision and utilization of multiple services.[555, 556] While effective delivery of health, child welfare, and educational services improves the lives of families who are able to access them, integration of the social services and health systems has been shown to further improve access to and provision of necessary services.[557-560]

System-wide education and training

Recovery-oriented systems of care will ensure that concepts of recovery and wellness are foundational elements of curricula, certification, licensure, accreditation and testing mechanisms. The workforce also requires continual training, at every level, to reinforce the tenets of recovery-oriented systems of care.

Educational interventions have been shown to improve physician performance and patient identification and outcomes of care.[561,562] A meta-analysis of disease management, which incorporated case management, found that improved disease control was associated with education of providers.[563] Furthermore, Bukstein et al. (2005) found that continuing education is essential to providing care that is based on the latest clinical and service interventions.[564]

Ongoing monitoring and outreach

Recovery-oriented systems of care will provide ongoing monitoring and feedback with assertive outreach efforts to promote continual participation, re-motivation and reengagement.

Models of ongoing monitoring and early reintervention occupy a central role in the long-term management of chronic medical conditions.[565-568] Accumulating evidence suggests that many cases of substance use problems and disorders should be continually monitored and are best treated with "the same type and level of ongoing clinical support as other chronic illnesses."[569]

The evidence shows that it is necessary to continuously evaluate and maintain connections with individuals in recovery, and by doing so, individuals at risk for relapse can reenter treatment at an earlier point of relapse.[570] In general, about 50–60 percent of patients begin reusing within 6 months of treatment cessation; therefore, it is essential for ongoing monitoring and outreach to be conducted.[571-574] Individuals who are readmitted sooner after relapse have better short-and long-term abstinence, improved outcome measures for employment and criminality, and lower associated substance use problems.[575, 576]

Outcomes driven

Recovery-oriented systems of care will be guided by recovery-based process and outcome measures. These measures will be developed in collaboration with individuals in recovery. Outcome measures will reflect the long-term global effects of the recovery process on the individual, family and community, not just remission of biomedical symptoms. Outcomes will be measurable and include benchmarks of quality-of-life changes.

There are several entities and projects focused on measuring substance use disorders process measures and outcomes. Examples include:

- Network for the Improvement of Addiction Treatment (NIATx; http://www.niatx.net), a partnership between the Robert Wood Johnson Foundation's Paths to Recovery program, the Center for Substance Abuse Treatment's Strengthening Treatment Access and Retention (STAR) program, NIDA, and a number of independent addictions treatment organizations, and
- Washington Circle (http://www.washingtoncircle.org), a policy group on performance measurement for care of substance use problems and disorders

These entities have independently developed process of care and performance measures aimed to improve treatment access and retention for individuals with substance use problems and disorders.

NIATx aims to improve access to treatment through its four process measures:

1. Average time from first request to first client treatment session;
2. "No Shows," which measures the number of patients who do not keep an appointment;
3. "Admissions," which counts the number of unduplicated client admissions by provider; and
4. "Continuation," which measures of the number of clients who stay engaged in treatment.

Washington Circle has and continues to develop performance measures in four domains of the process of care:

1. Prevention/Education
2. Recognition
3. Treatment
   a. Initiation of alcohol and other plan services
   b. Linkage of detoxification, alcohol, and other drug plans
   c. Treatment engagement
   d. Interventions for family members and significant others
4. Maintenance of treatment effects

Many large-scale longitudinal outcome studies have been conducted that examine various indicators of life changes, including substance use behavior, criminal behavior, education, employment, health, and social support. Examples of these data collection and outcome evaluation efforts include the Drug Abuse Treatment Outcome Study (DATOS) conducted by NIDA, the National Treatment Improvement Evaluation Study (NTIES) by SAMHSA, the Alcohol and Drug Services Study (ADSS) by SAMHSA, and the California Outcome Study using the California Drug and Alcohol Treatment Assessment (CALDATA) by the State of California. These data sets examine the impact of treatment and behavior change processes on quality of life outcomes.

Research based

Recovery-oriented systems of care will be informed by research. Additional research on individuals in recovery, recovery venues and the processes of recovery, including cultural and spiritual aspects, is essential.

Research will be supplemented by the experiences of people in recovery.

This white paper is a critical first step in examining how the research relates to the principles of recovery and systems of care elements and identifies where additional research is needed.

Adequately and flexibly financed.

Recovery-oriented systems of care will be adequately financed to permit access to a full continuum of services, ranging from detoxification and treatment to continuing care and recovery support. In addition, funding will be sufficiently flexible to permit unbundling of services, enabling the establishment of a customized array of services that can evolve over time in support of an individual's recovery.

Pooling of funding may reduce problems associated with fragmented funding and separate service systems. Pooled funding also may improve service coordination within and between different organizations and networks and may work to expand access to and provision of services.[577] Additionally, States and service facilities can utilize creative financing mechanisms to provide and reimburse for recovery-oriented services. For example, Michigan's State agencies have organized multiple funding sources to provide integrated community mental health and primary medical care, and have improved access to these services.[578]

Voucher programs provide people seeking drug and alcohol treatment and recovery support services with a funding mechanism to pay for a range of unbundled community-based services. Many States, through the Access to Recovery grant program, have implemented voucher programs to improve Access to Recovery support services and promote patient choice in service provision.

8. Research Supporting the Implementation of Recovery-Oriented Services and Systems of Care

While many States (e.g., Connecticut, Georgia, Massachusetts, Michigan, New Jersey, New York, and Oregon) and cities (e.g., Philadelphia) are in the process of reforming their systems to implement recovery-oriented systems of care, there are few publications in peer-reviewed journals that describe the effectiveness of this systems change for individuals with substance use problems and disorders. However, there are several published articles in peer-reviewed journals that discuss the implementation and delivery of recovery-oriented services in the mental health system. This section discusses the available peer-reviewed literature focusing on the delivery of recovery-oriented services and the implementation of recovery-oriented systems of care in the addictions and mental health fields.

In 2000, the State of Connecticut embarked on transforming its system of publicly funded behavioral health care into a system that is recovery-oriented and culturally responsive. In 2002, Connecticut was the first State that incorporated recovery as the overarching aim of its publicly funded system of care.[579] The initiative targeted the statewide system of care as a whole instead of supplementing the existing system with recovery-oriented elements.[580] The Connecticut initiative involved several interrelated steps occurring over several years:

1. Developing core values and principles based on the input of people in recovery;
2. Establishing a conceptual framework based on this vision of recovery;
3. Building workforce competencies and skills through training, education, and consultation;
4. Changing programs and service structures;
5. Aligning fiscal and administrative policies in support of recovery; and
6. Monitoring, evaluating, and adjusting the efforts.

Two peer-reviewed articles describe the implementation efforts of the Connecticut system. A 2005 article in *Psychiatric Rehabilitation Journal* outlines the results of a recovery self-assessment implemented in Connecticut, which gauged perceptions of the degree to which programs implement recovery-oriented practices.[581] In this article, O'Connell et al. provide a statewide assessment of recovery-oriented practices in agencies. Results indicated that mental health professionals, persons in recovery, and family members "generally agreed that their agencies were providing services that are consistent with a recovery orientation."[582] A 2007 article in *Psychiatric Rehabilitation Journal* provides evaluative details on the implementation of the early stages of the initiative.[583] Two themes are discussed:

1. Recovery does not refer to any specific service, intervention, or support (which can be more or less recovery oriented) but to what people with psychiatric disabilities or addiction do themselves in order to manage their illness and/or get their lives back.
2. Recovery cannot be an "add-on" to existing services, supports, or systems. The focus of transformation needs to be on changing and realigning current policies, practices, procedures, services, and supports to be oriented toward, and effective in, promoting recovery.

In 2004, Philadelphia created the city's Department of Behavioral Health and Mental Retardation Services, which combined the Community Behavioral Health Office, the Office of Mental Health, and the Coordinating Office for Drug and Alcohol Abuse Programs into an integrated behavioral health care system.[584] The systems transformation in Philadelphia included numerous stakeholders in the process, including recovering people and their families, in developing a vision for the Philadelphia system. This vision and mission of Philadelphia was to create an integrated system that "promotes long-term recovery, resiliency, self-determination, and a meaningful life in the community," which shifted the values of the system from the "interventions of professional experts to the experience and needs of recovering individuals and their families."[585, p.36] Relationships between service practitioners, service consumers, the department, and local services providers shifted to partnerships based on mutual respect and collaborations. Additionally, "recovery representation" was emphasized at all levels of the system to "affirm that recovery is a living reality in the City of Philadelphia."[586] Practices of delivery services were changed to improve care delivery and focus on recovery. As discussed by White (2007) in his description of the recovery revolution in Philadelphia, in 10 service areas changes to the system occurred. These areas are the following: engagement, assessment, retention, role of client, service relationship, clinical care, service dose/duration, service delivery sites, post treatment checkups and support, and attitude toward readmission.[587]

Finally, Philadelphia worked with multiple constituents to plan and implement changes in funding and regulatory policies, which are critical to effectively implement and sustain the behavioral health system, and to focus its regulatory and policy reform on recovery. Philadelphia has focused on "providing regulatory relief (reducing duplicative and excessive regulatory requirements), generating more recovery-focused regulatory standards, shifting the focus of program monitoring from one of policing to one of consultation and support, generating new Request for Proposals for recovery-focused service initiatives, and exploring models for long-term funding of recovery support services."[588]

The State of Massachusetts, through its Departments of Mental Health and Public Health, designed a collaborative model to provide a comprehensive integrated service system for persons with co-occurring substance use problems and disorders and serious mental illness for the private and public sectors. Barreira, Espey, Fishbein, Moran, and Flannery (2000) describe the design phase of Massachusetts' integrated system and provide lessons learned and outcomes for developing the system, but the implementation of the initiative has not yet been published.[589] Specifically, the authors discuss utilizing a collaborative framework, which includes involving the key stakeholders, to foster change and buy-in for the system. The collaborative and consensus-building process builds on evidence-based practices and best practices, builds on organizational strengths, and is sensitive to barriers to change (e.g., differing philosophies, regulatory processes, clinical and administrative traditions and policies, resistance to change) and collaboration. Massachusetts also discovered that "providing a voice for stakeholders who are parties in designing change" and "developing consensus on a framework of care that all groups endorse" so funding resources are not seen as being taken from one system to another were critical for the collaborative process to succeed and the integrated framework to be implemented.[590]

Jacobson and Curtis, in a 2000 Psychiatric Rehabilitation Journal article, outline how the concept of recovery is being implemented in the policies and practices of several State mental health systems and review specific strategies that States, including Wisconsin, Ohio, Vermont, and Nebraska, are using to implement recovery principles into their mental health systems.[591] Most of the State systems reviewed begin their systems' transformation with the development of vision statements in consensus workgroups and task forces, renaming programs, and applying strategies for operationalizing recovery-oriented services. Both programmatic and administrative strategies are being adopted to implement recovery-oriented services; they include education, consumer and family involvement, support for consumer-operated services, emphasis on relapse prevention and management, incorporation of crisis planning and advance directives, implementing stigma reduction initiatives, innovations in contracting and financing mechanisms, definition and measurement of outcomes, and reviewing and revising key policies. In this article, while Jacobson and Curtis do not specifically review activities that occur across different service systems, they discuss the importance of involving a variety of stakeholders in the systems-change effort and of recovery education initiatives and the destigmatization that is occurring across workers in different disciplinary backgrounds, consumers, family members, and administrators. They further state that the concept of recovery must look beyond the service provider and the mental health system.

Modification of Philadelphia Department of Behavioral Health and Mental Retardation Services Service System and Clinical Practice to be More Recovery Oriented (White, 2007, pp. 36-27)

1. *Engagement*: Greater focus on early identification via outreach and community education; emphasis on removing personal and environmental obstacles to recovery; shift in responsibility for motivation to change from the client to service provider; loosening of admission criteria; renewed focus on the quality of the service relationship.
2. *Assessment*: Greater use of global and strength-based assessment instruments and interview protocol; shift from assessment as an intake activity to assessment as a continuing activity focused on the developmental stages of recovery.
3. *Retention*: Increased focus on service retention and decreasing premature service disengagement; use of outreach workers, recovery coaches, and advocates to reduce rates of client disengagement and administrative discharge.
4. *Role of Client*: Shift toward philosophy of choice rather than prescription of pathways and styles of recovery; greater client authority and decision-making within the service relationship; emphasis on empowering clients to self-manage their own recoveries.
5. *Service Relationship*: Service relationships are less hierarchical with counselor serving more as ongoing recovery consultant than professional expert; more a stance of "How can I help you?" than "This is what you must do."
6. *Clinical Care*: Greater accountability for delivery of services that are evidence-based, gender-sensitive, culturally competent, and trauma informed; greater integration of professional counseling and peer-based recovery support services; considerable emphasis on understanding and modifying each client's recovery environment; use of formal recovery circles (recovery support network development).
7. *Service Dose/Duration*: Dose and duration of total services will increase while number and duration of acute care episodes will decline; emphasis shifts from crisis stabilization to ongoing recovery coaching; great value placed in continuity of contact in a primary recovery support relationship over time

8. *Service Delivery Sites*: Emphasis on transfer of learning from institutional to natural environments; greater emphasis on home-based and neighborhood-based service delivery; greater use of community organization skills to build or help revitalize indigenous recovery supports where they are absent or weak.
9. *Post-treatment Checkups and Support*: Emphasis on recovery resource development (e.g., supporting alumni groups and expansion/diversification of local recovery support groups); assertive linkage to communities of recovery; face-to-face, telephone-based, or Internet-based post-treatment monitoring and support; stage-appropriate recovery education; and, when needed, early re-intervention.
10. *Attitude toward Re-admission*: Returning clients are welcomed (not shamed); emphasis on transmitting principles and strategies of chronic disease management; focus on enhancement of recovery maintenance skills rather than recycling through standard programs focused on recovery initiation; emphasis on enhancing peer-based recovery supports and minimizing need for high-intensity professional services.

In a 2004 article that outlines the complementary nature of evidence-based practices and recovery in a service system, Solomon and Stanhope describe the profound changes required at the systems level for the implementation of evidence-based practices and recovery-oriented services.[592] The authors trace the integration of a recovery orientation into the Ohio Department of Mental Health. In 1993, Ohio started the process to transform its system. The first step of the transformation was to have a dialog with providers, consumers, and family members to explore the mental health recovery process and prepare a report outlining the stages of the process. The stages were integrated into a framework for implementing recovery-oriented practices, which included clinical care, peer and family support, facilitation of employment, empowerment, stigma reduction, community involvement, access to resources, and education. By offering grants to localities, Ohio helped localities transform their mental health systems through establishing recovery centers and recovery management plans within agencies. "The Ohio recovery model is an example of tailoring a recovery vision to the specific needs of consumers and implementing change through financial incentives." [593, p.318] Other States, including California, Massachusetts, New York, and Washington, have written recovery principles within their State managed care contracts. These principles "require that organizations contract with providers who pursue recovery-oriented services, including consumer-operated services, and that consumers have an advisory role on managed care organization boards."[594, p.319]

Conclusion

This white paper examines the research that supports the principles of recovery and systems of care elements as defined by the National Summit on Recovery. The author identified findings in more than 375 studies that supported the framework, principles, elements, and implementation of recovery-oriented services and systems. This document is intended to serve as a starting point for further examination of recovery research. Additionally, it provides States, communities, and organizations that are developing and implementing recovery-oriented services and systems with evidence that supports services and systems improvements based on recovery-oriented approaches.

While many of the principles and systems elements are easily supported by existing literature in the addictions field, research supporting others was more difficult to find. In some circumstances, they were supported by literature outside of addictions research, primarily through the mental health and public health research fields. What follows is a brief synopsis of the research that was found to support the principles of recovery and systems of care elements and a listing of the fields from which the information was derived.

Extensive research has been conducted in the addictions field to support the following principles and systems elements:

- There are many pathways to recovery;
- Recovery exists on a continuum of improved health and wellness;
- Recovery is supported by peers and allies;
- Recovery is a reality;
- Inclusive of family and other ally involvement;
- Individualized and comprehensive services across the lifespan;
- Continuing care part of the continuity of care element;
- Partnership-consultant relationships;
- Responsiveness to personal belief systems;
- Commitment to peer recovery support services;
- Integrated services; and
- Ongoing monitoring and outreach.

The following principles and systems elements were supported by a modest amount of research from the addictions field:

- Recovery is self-directed and empowering;
- Recovery involves a personal recognition of the need for change and transformation;
- Recovery emerges from hope and gratitude;
- Recovery involves addressing discrimination and transcending shame and stigma;
- Recovery involves (re)joining and (re)building a life in the community;
- Systems anchored in the community;
- Strength-based; and
- Outcomes driven.

The following principles and systems elements were supported by limited addictions research, but were grounded in literature from the general public health and mental health fields:

- Recovery has cultural dimensions;
- Person-centered;
- Continuity of care;
- Culturally responsive;

- Inclusion of the voices and experiences of recovering individuals and their families; and
- System-wide education and training.

The following principles were supported by a minimal amount of research in the addictions, mental health, and public health research fields:

- Recovery is holistic;
- Recovery involves a process of healing and self-redefinition; and
- Adequately and flexibly financed.

In relation to the process-and outcomes-driven systems element, it should be noted that large-scale, longitudinal studies have been conducted that measure quality-of-life outcomes for individuals with substance use problems and disorders. However, this systems element points to the importance of examining long-term global effects of the recovery process on the individual, family, and community, while also studying the process of care and implementing continuous quality improvement mechanisms to improve treatment access and retention. Additionally, this element suggests that process and outcome measures should be developed in collaboration with individuals in recovery. Although the addictions research community includes some researchers in recovery, this element suggests broader inclusion of the voices of individuals in recovery in developing outcome measures.

Finally, this paper identifies areas where there are modest amounts of addictions research related to recovery. Limited literature on the conceptual framework of recovery-oriented systems of care exists, but even less research is available on the implementation and outcomes of recovery-oriented services and systems for those with substance use problems and disorders. By providing this baseline assessment and the associated gaps in the research, future research agendas can be better informed.

REFERENCES

[1] Center for Substance Abuse Treatment. (2005). *National Summit on Recovery: Conference Report.* DHHS Publication No. (SMA) 07-4276. Rockville, MD: Substance Abuse and Mental Health Services Administration.

[2] Anthony, W. A. (2000). A recovery-oriented service system: setting some system level standards. *Psychiatric Rehabilitation Journal*, *24(*2), 159–168.

[3] O'Connell, M., Tondora, J., Croog, G., Evans, A. & Davidson, L. (2005). From rhetoric to routine: Assessing perceptions of recovery-oriented practices in a state mental health and addiction system. *Psychiatric Rehabilitation Journal*, 28(4), 378–386.

[4] Gagne, C., White, W. & Anthony, W. A. (2007) Recovery: A common vision for the fields of mental health and addictions. *Psychiatric Rehabilitation Journal*, *31*(1), 32-37.

[5] Ibid.

[6] Friedmann, P. D., Hendrickson, J. C., Gerstein, D. R., & Zhang, Z. (2004). The effect of matching comprehensive services to patients' needs on drug use improvement in addiction treatment. *Addiction*, 99(8), 962–972,

[7] Simpson, D. D., Joe, G. W., Greener, J. M. & Rowan-Szal, G. A. (2000). Modeling year 1 outcomes with treatment process and post-treatment social influences. *Substance Use and Misuse*, *35*, 1911–1930.

[8] Joe, G. W., Broome, K. M., Rowan-Szal, G. A. & Simpson, D. D. (2002). Measuring patient attributes and engagement in treatment. *Journal of Substance Abuse Treatment*, *22*(4), 183–196

[9] Hser, Y. I., Evans, E., Huang, D. & Anglin, D. M. (2004). Relationship between drug treatment services, retention, and outcomes. *Psychiatric Services*, *55*(7), 767–774.

[10] French, M. T., McGeary, K. A., Chitwood, D. D. & McCoy, C. B. (2000). Chronic illicit drug use, health services utilization and the cost of medical care. *Social Science & Medicine*, *50*, 1703–1713.

[11] French, M. T., Salome, H. J., Sindelar, J. L. & McLellan, A. T. (2002). Benefit-cost analysis of addiction treatment: Methodological guidelines and empirical application using the DATCAP and ASI. *Health Services Research*, *37*, 433–455.

[12] Hser, Y. I., Hoffman, V., Grella, C. E. & Anglin, M. D. (2001). A 33-year follow-up of narcotics addicts. *Archives of General Psychiatry*, *58*, 503–508.

[13] Etheridge, R. M, Craddock, S. G., Dunteman, G. H. & Hubbard, R. L. (1995). Treatment services in two national studies of community-based drug abuse treatment programs. *Journal of Substance Abuse*, *7*(1), 9–26.

[14] Salome, H. J., French, M. T., Miller, M. & McLellan, A. T. (2003). Estimating the client costs of addiction treatment: First findings from the client drug abuse treatment cost analysis program (Client DATCAP). *Drug and Alcohol Dependence*, *71*, 195–206.

[15] Simpson, D. D. & Sells, S. B. (1974). Patterns of multiple drug abuse: 1969-1971. *International Journal of Addictions*, *9*, 301–314.

[16] Simpson, D. D., Joe, G. W. & Rowan-Szal, G. A. (1997). Drug abuse treatment retention and process effects on follow-up outcomes. *Drug and Alcohol Dependence*, *47*, 227–235.

[17] Simpson, D. D., Joe, G. W., Fletcher, B. W., Hubbard, R. L. & Anglin, M. D. (1999). A national evaluation of treatment outcomes for cocaine dependence. *Archives of General Psychiatry*, *56*, 507–514.

[18] Simpson, D. D. (2004). A conceptual framework for drug treatment process and outcomes. *Journal of Substance Abuse Treatment*, *27*, 99–121.

[19] McLellan, A. T., Lewis, D. C., O'Brien, C. P. & Kleber, H. D. (2000). Drug dependence, a chronic medical illness: Implications for treatment, insurance, and outcomes evaluation. *Journal of the American Medical Association*, *284*(13), 1689–1695.

[20] McLellan, A. T., Woody, G. E., Metzger, D., McKay, J., Alterman, A. I. & O'Brien, C. P. (1996). Evaluating the effectiveness of addiction treatments: Reasonable expectations, appropriate comparisons. *Milbank Quarterly*, *74*(1), 51–85.

[21] Simpson, D. D. & Brown, B. S. (Eds.) (1999). Treatment process and outcome studies from DATOS [Special issue]. *Drug and Alcohol Dependence*, *57*.

[22] Simpson, D. D. & Curry, S. J. (Eds.) (1997). Drug Abuse Treatment Outcome Study (DATOS) [Special issue]. *Psychology of Addictive Behaviors*, *11*.

[23] Simpson, D. D. & Sells, S. B. (1982). Effectiveness of treatment for drug abuse: An overview of the DARP research program. *Advances in Alcohol and Substance Abuse*, *2*, 7–29.

[24] Lamb, S., Greenlick, M. R. & McCarty, D. (1998). *Bridging the gap between practice and research: Forging partnerships with community-based drug and alcohol treatment.* Washington, DC: National Academy Press.

[25] Leshner, A. I. (1997). Drug abuse and addiction treatment research. The next generation. *Archives of General Psychiatry*, *54*, 691–694.

[26] McLellan, A. T., Lewis, D. C., O'Brien, C. P. & Kleber, H. D. (2000). Drug dependence, a chronic medical illness: Implications for treatment, insurance, and outcomes evaluation. *Journal of the American Medical Association*, *284*, 1689–1695.

[27] Haggerty, J. L., Reid, R. J., Freeman, G. K., Starfield, B. H., Adair, C. E. & McKendry, R. (2003). Continuity of care: A multidisciplinary review. *British Medical Journal*, *327*, 1219–1221.

[28] Humphreys, K., Moos, R. H. & Finney, J. W. (1995). Two pathways out of drinking problems without professional treatment. *Addictive Behaviors*, *20*(4), 427–441.

[29] White, W. L., Boyle, M. & Loveland, D. (2002). Alcoholism/addiction as a chronic disease: From rhetoric to clinical reality. *Alcoholism Treatment Quarterly*, *20*(3/4), 107–130.

[30] Laudet, A. B., Savage, R. & Mahmood, D. (2002). Pathways to long-term recovery: A preliminary investigation. *Journal of Psychoactive Drugs*, *34*(3), 305–311.

[31] Hser, Y., Longshore, D. & Anglin, M. D. (2007). The life course perspective on drug use: A conceptual framework for understanding drug use trajectories. *Evaluation Review*, *31*(6), 515–547.

[32] Ibid.

[33] Ibid, 517.

[34] Babor, T. F., Stenius, K. & Romelsjo, A. (2008), Alcohol and drug treatment systems in public health perspective: Mediators and moderators of population effects. *International Journal of Methods in Psychiatric Research*, *17*(S1), S50–S59.

[35] Ibid.

[36] Ibid.

[37] Ibid.

[38] Ibid.

[39] Minkoff, K. & Cline, C. A. (2004). Changing the world: The design and implementation of comprehensive continuous integrated systems of care for individuals with co-occurring disorders. *Psychiatric Clinics of North America*, *27*(4), 727–743.

[40] Minkoff, K. & Cline, C. A. (2004). Changing the world: The design and implementation of comprehensive continuous integrated systems of care for individuals with co-occurring disorders. *Psychiatric Clinics of North America*, *27*(4), 727–743.

[41] Frese, F. F., Stanley, J., Kress, K. & Vogel-Scibilia, S. (2001). Integrating evidence-based practices and the recovery model. *Psychiatric Services*, *52*(11), 1462–1468.

[42] Jacobson, N. & Greenley, D. (2001). What is recovery? A conceptual model and explication. *Psychiatric Services*, *52*, 482–485.

[43] Jacobson, N. & Curtis, L. (2000). Recovery as policy in mental health services: Strategies emerging from the states. *Psychiatric Rehabilitation Journal*, *23*(4), 333–341.

[44] Solomon, P. & Stanhope, V. (2004). Recovery: Expanding the vision of evidence-based practice. *Brief Treatment and Crisis Intervention*, *4*(4), 311–321.

[45] Anthony, W. A. (1993). Recovery from mental illness: The guiding vision of the mental health service system in the 1990s. *Psychiatric Rehabilitation Journal*, *16*(4), 11–23.
[46] Anthony, W. A. (2000). A recovery-oriented service system: Setting some system level standards. *Psychiatric Rehabilitation Journal*, *24*(2), 159–168.
[47] Anthony, W. A. (2000). A recovery-oriented service system: Setting some system level standards. *Psychiatric Rehabilitation Journal*, *24*(2), 159–168.
[48] Ibid.
[49] Jacobson, N. & Curtis, L. (2000).
[50] Barton, R. (1998). The rehabilitation-recovery paradigm: A statement of philosophy for a public mental health system. *Psychiatric Rehabilitation Skills*., *2*(2), 171–187.
[51] Ibid, 177.
[52] National Institute on Drug Abuse. (1999; reprinted 2000). *Principles of drug addiction treatment: A research based guide* (NIH Publication No. 00–4180). Bethesda, MD: National Institutes of Health.
[53] Laudet, A. B., Savage, R. & Mahmood, D. (2002).
[54] Venner, K. L., Matzger, H., Forcehimes, A. A., Moos, R. H., Feldstein, S. W. Willenbring, M. L. et al. (2006). Course of recovery from alcoholism. *Alcoholism, Clinical and Experimental Research*, *30*, 1079–1090.
[55] Laudet, A. B., Savage, R. & Mahmood, D. (2002).
[56] Havassy, B. E., Hall, S. M. & Wasserman, D. A. (1991). Social support and relapse: Commonalities among alcoholics, opiate users, and cigarette smokers. *Addictive Behaviors*, *16*, 235–246.
[57] Sobell, L. C., Sobell, M. B., Toneatto, T. & Leo, G. I. (1993). Severely dependent alcohol abusers may be vulnerable to alcohol cues in television programs. *Journal of Studies on Alcohol*, *54*, 85–91.
[58] Fillmore, K. M., Grant, M., Hartka, E., Johnstone, B. M., Sawyer, S. M. & Speiglman, R. et al. (1988). Collaborative longitudinal research on alcohol problems. *British Journal of Addictions*, *83*, 441–444.
[59] Sobell, L. C., Sobell, M. B., Toneatto, T. & Leo, G. I. (1993). What triggers the resolution of alcohol problems without treatment. *Alcoholism, Clinical and Experimental Research*, *17*, 217–224.
[60] Cunningham, J. A., Sobell, L. C., Sobell, M. B. & Kapur, G. (1995). Resolution from alcohol problems with and without treatment: Reasons for change. *Journal of Substance Abuse*, *7*(3), 365–72.
[61] Cunningham, J. A. (1999). Untreated remissions from drug use: The predominant pathway. *Addictive Behaviors*, *24*, 267–270.
[62] Cunningham, J. A. (1999). Resolving alcohol-related problems with and without treatment: The effects of different problem criteria. *Journal of Studies on Alcohol*, *60*, 463–466.
[63] Sobell, L. C., Cunningham, J. A. & Sobell, M. B. (1996). Recovery from alcohol problems with and without treatment: Prevalence in two population surveys. *American Journal of Public Health*, *86*, 966–972.
[64] Sobell, L. C., Ellingstad, T. P. & Sobell, M. B. (2000). Natural recovery from alcohol and drug problems: Methodological review of the research with suggestions for future directions. *Addiction*, *95*, 749–764.
[65] Ibid.

[66] Sobell, L. C., Sobell, M. B., Toneatto, T. et al (1993).

[67] Sobell, L. C., Cunningham, J. A. & Sobell, M. B. (1996).

[68] Larimer, M. E. & Kilmer, J. R. (2000). Natural history. In G. Zernig, A. Saria, M. Kurz & S. S. O'Malley (Eds.), *Handbook of alcoholism* (13–28). Boca Raton, FL: CRC Press.

[69] Latkin, C. A., Knowlton, A. R., Hoover, D. & Mandell, W. (1999). Drug network characteristics as a predictor of cessation of drug use among adult injection drug users: A prospective study. *The American Journal of Drug and Alcohol Abuse*, *25*(3), 463–473.

[70] Weisner, C., Matzger, H. & Kaskutas, L. A. (2003). How important is treatment? One-year outcomes of treated and untreated alcohol-dependent individuals. *Addiction*, *98*, 901–911.

[71] Bischof, G., Rumpf, H. J., Hapke, U., Meyer, C. & John, U. (2001). Factors influencing remission from alcohol dependence without formal help in a representative population sample. *Addiction*, *96*, 1327–1336.

[72] Russell, M., Peirce, R. S., Chan, A. W. K., Wieczorek, W. F., Moscato, B. S. & Nochajski, T. H. (2001). Natural recovery in a community-based sample of alcoholics: Study design and descriptive data. *Substance Use and Misuse*, *36*(11), 1417–1441.

[73] Weisner, C., Matzger, H. & Kaskutas, L. A. (2003).

[74] Bischof, G., Rumpf, H. J., Hapke, U., Meyer, C. & John, U. (2001).

[75] Russell, M., Peirce, R. S., Chan, A. W. K., Wieczorek, W. F., Moscato, B. S. & Nochajski, T. H. (2001).

[76] Granfield, R. & Cloud, W. (2001). Social context and "natural recovery": The role of social capital in the resolution of drug-associated problems. *Substance Use and Misuse*, *36*, 1543–1570.

[77] Ibid, 1566.

[78] Etheridge, R. M, Craddock, S. G., Dunteman, G. H. & Hubbard, R. L. (1995).

[79] Simpson, D. D. & Sells, S. B. (1974).

[80] Simpson, D. D., Joe, G. W. & Rowan-Szal, G. A. (1997).

[81] Simpson, D. D., Joe, G. W., Fletcher, B. W., Hubbard, R. L. & Anglin, M. D. (1999).

[82] French, M. T., McGeary, K. A., Chitwood, D. D. & McCoy, C. B. (2000). Chronic illicit drug use, health services utilization and the cost of medical care. *Social Science & Medicine*, *50*, 1703–1713.

[83] French, M. T., Salome, H. J., Sindelar, J. L. & McLellan, A. T. (2002). Benefit-cost analysis of addiction treatment: Methodological guidelines and empirical application using the DATCAP and ASI. *Health Services Research*, *37*, 433-455.

[84] Hser, Y. I., Hoffman, V., Grella, C. E. & Anglin, M. D. (2001). A 33-year follow-up of narcotics addicts. *Archives of General Psychiatry*, *58*, 503–508.

[85] Salome, H. J., French, M. T., Miller, M. & McLellan, A. T. (2003). Estimating the client costs of addiction treatment: First findings from the client drug abuse treatment cost analysis program (Client DATCAP). *Drug and Alcohol Dependence*, *71*, 195–206.

[86] Cunningham, J. A., Koski-Jannes, A. & Toneatto, T. (1999). Why do people stop their drug use? Results from a general population sample. *Contemporary Drug Problems*, *26*, 695–710.

[87] Cunningham, J. A., Lin, E., Ross, H. E. & Walsh, G. W. (2000). Factors associated with untreated remissions from alcohol abuse or dependence. *Addictive Behaviors*, *25*, 317–321.

[88] Laudet, A. B., Savage, R. & Mahmood, D. (2002).

[89] Miller, W. R. & Longabaugh, R. (2002). Summary and conclusions. In T. F. Babor & F. K. Del Boca (Eds.), *Treatment matching in alcoholism*. Cambridge, UK: Cambridge University Press.

[90] Ouimette, P. C., Moos, R. H. & Finney, J. W. (1998). Influence of outpatient treatment and 12-step group involvement on one-year substance abuse treatment outcomes. *Journal of Studies on Alcohol*, *59*, 513–522.

[91] Scott, C. K., Dennis, M. L. & Foss, M. A. (2005). Utilizing recovery management checkups to shorten the cycle of relapse, treatment reentry, and recovery. *Drug and Alcohol Dependence*, *78*, 325–338.

[92] Florentine, R. (1999). After drug treatment: Are 12-step programs effective in maintaining abstinence? *American Journal of Drug and Alcohol Abuse*, *25*, 93–116.

[93] Miller, N. S., Ninonuevo, F. G., Klamen, D. L., Hoffmann, N. G. & Smith, D. E. (1997). Integration of treatment and posttreatment variables in predicting results of abstinence-based outpatient treatment after one year. *Journal of Psychoactive Drugs*, *29*, 239–248.

[94] McKellar, J., Kelly, J., Harris, A. & Moos, R. (2006). Pretreatment and during treatment risk factors for dropout among patients with substance use disorders. *Addictive Behaviors*, *31*(3), 450–60. Epub 2005 Jun 23.

[95] Tonigan, J. S., Miller, W. R. & Conners, G. J. (2001). The search for meaning in life as a predictor of alcoholism treatment outcome. In R. Longabaugh & P. W. Wirtz (Eds.), *Project MATCH Monograph Series: Vol. 8. Project MATCH hypotheses: Results and causal chain analysis* (154–165). Bethesda, MD: National Institute on Alcohol Abuse and Alcoholism.

[96] Connors, G. J., Tonigan, J. S. & Miller, W. R. (2001). A longitudinal model of intake symptomatology, AA participation and outcome: Retrospective study of the project MATCH outpatient and aftercare samples. *Journal of Studies on Alcohol*, *62*, 817–825.

[97] Johnson, N. P. & Chappel, J. N. (1994). Using AA and other 12-step programs more effectively. *Journal of Substance Abuse Treatment*, *11*(2), 137–142.

[98] Khantzian, E. J. & Mack, J. E. (1994). How AA works and why it's important for clinicians to understand. *Journal of Substance Abuse Treatment*, *11*(2), 77–92.

[99] Laudet, A. B., Savage, R. & Mahmood, D. (2002).

[100] Scott, C. K., Dennis, M. L. & Foss, M. A. (2005).

[101] Tonigan, J. S., Miller, W. R. & Conners, G. J. (2001).

[102] Connors, G. J., Tonigan, J. S. & Miller, W. R. (2001). A longitudinal model of intake symptomatology, AA participation and outcome: Retrospective study of the project MATCH outpatient and aftercare samples. *Journal of Studies on Alcohol*, *62*, 817–825.

[103] Johnson, N. P. & Chappel, J. N. (1994). Using AA and other 12-step programs more effectively. *Journal of Substance Abuse Treatment*, *11*(2), 137–142.

[104] Tonigan, J. S., Miller, W. R. & Conners, G. J. (2001).

[105] Connors, G. J., Tonigan, J. S. & Miller, W. R. (2001). A longitudinal model of intake symptomatology, AA participation and outcome: Retrospective study of the project MATCH outpatient and aftercare samples. *Journal of Studies on Alcohol*, *62*, 817–825.

[106] Johnson, N. P. & Chappel, J. N. (1994). Using AA and other 12-step programs more effectively. *Journal of Substance Abuse Treatment*, *11*(2), 137–142.
[107] Kreek, M. J. & Vocci, F. J. (2002). History and current status of opioid maintenance treatments: Blending conference session. *Journal of Substance Abuse Treatment*, *23*(2), 93–105.
[108] National Consensus Development Panel on Effective Medical Treatment of Opiate Addiction. (1998). Effective medical treatment of opiate addiction. *JAMA*, *280*, 1936–1943.
[109] Doty, P., Kasper, J. & Litvak, S. (1996). Consumer-directed models of personal care: Lessons from Medicaid. *Milbank Quarterly*, *74*(3), 377–409.
[110] Tilly, J. & Wiener, J. (2001a). Consumer-directed home and community services programs in eight states: Policy issues for older people and government. *Journal of Aging and Social Policy*, *12*(4), 1–2.
[111] Tilly, J. & Wiener, J. (2001b). *Consumer-directed home and community services: Policy issues*. Washington, DC: The Urban Institute.
[112] Foster, L., Brown, R., Phillips, B., Schore, J., Lepidus, R. & Carlson, B. (2003). Improving the quality of Medicaid personal assistance through consumer direction. *Health Affairs Web Exclusive* [serial online], Mar 26. Retrieved from http://www.healthaffairs.org/WebExclusives/FosterWebExcl032603.htm.
[113] Lorig, K. R. & Holman, H. (2003). Self-management education: History, definition, outcomes, and mechanisms. *Annals of Behavioral Medicine*, *26*, 1–7.
[114] Lorig, K. R., Ritter, P., Stewart, A. L., Sobel, D. S., Brown, B. W. & Bandura, A. et al. (2001). Chronic disease self-management program: 2-year health status and health care utilization outcomes. *Medical Care*, *39*, 1217–1223.
[115] Shoor, S. & Lorig, K. R. (2002). Self-care and the doctor-patient relationship. *Medical Care*, *40*, 1140–1144.
[116] Institute of Medicine. (2006). *Improving the quality of health care for mental and substance use conditions*. Washington, DC: National Academy of Sciences.
[117] Samet, J. H., Rollnick, S. & Barnes, H. (1996). Beyond CAGE: A brief clinical approach after detection of substance abuse. *Archives of Internal Medicine*, *156*, 2287–2293.
[118] Morgenstern, J., Labouvie, E., McCrady, B. S., Kahler, C. W. & Frey, R. M. (1997). Affiliation with Alcoholics Anonymous after treatment: A study of its therapeutic effects and mechanisms of action. *Journal of Consulting and Clinical Psychology*, *65*, 768–777.
[119] Miller, W. R. (1996). Motivational interviewing: Research, practice, and puzzles. *Addictive Behaviors*, *21*, 835–842.
[120] Swanson, A. J., Pantalon, M. V. & Cohen, K. R. (1999). Motivational interviewing and treatment adherence among psychiatric and dually diagnosed patients. *Journal of Nervous and Mental Disease*, *187*, 630–635.
[121] Miller, W. R. & Rollnick, S. (1991). *Motivational interviewing: Preparing people to change addictive behavior*. New York: Guilford Press.
[122] Miller, W. R. & Rollnick, S. (2002). *Motivational interviewing: Preparing people for change* (2nd ed.). New York: Guilford Press.
[123] Rusch, N. & Corrigan, P. W. (2002). Motivational interviewing to improve insight and treatment adherence in schizophrenia. *Psychiatric Rehabilitation Journal*, *26*, 23–32.

[124] Miller, W. R. & Rollnick, S. (1991).
[125] Miller, W. R. & Rollnick, S. (2002).
[126] Venner, K. L., Matzger, H. & Forcehimes, A. A. et al. (2006).
[127] Maddux, J. F. & Desmond, D. P. (1986). Relapse and recovery in substance abuse careers. *NIDA Research Monograph*, *72*, 49–71.
[128] Miller, W. R. (1998). Researching the spiritual dimensions of alcohol and other drug problems. *Addiction*, 93, 979–990.
[129] Flynn, P. M., Joe, G. W., Broome, K. M., Simpson, D. D. & Brown, B. S. (2003). Recovery from opioid addiction in DATOS. *Journal of Substance Abuse Treatment*, *25*, 177–186.
[130] Drake, R. E., Wallach, M. A. & McGovern, M. P. (2005). Future directions in preventing relapse to substance abuse among clients with severe mental illnesses. *Psychiatric Services*, *56*, 1297–1302.
[131] Carpenter, K. M., Miele, G. M. & Hasin, D. S. (2002). Does motivation to change mediate the effect of DSM-IV substance use disorders on treatment utilization and substance use? *Addictive Behaviors*, *27*(2), 207–225.
[132] Joe, G. W., Simpson, D. D. & Broome, K. M. (1999). Retention and patient engagement models for different treatment modalities in DATOS. *Drug and Alcohol Dependence*, *57*, 113–125.
[133] Laudet, A. B., Morgen, K. & White, W. L. (2006). The role of social supports, spirituality, religiousness, life meaning and affiliation with 12-step fellowships in quality of life satisfaction among individuals in recovery from alcohol and drug problems. *Alcoholism Treatment Quarterly*, *24*, 33–73.
[134] Lowery, C. T. (1998). American Indian perspectives on addiction and recovery. *Health and Social Work*, *23*, 127–135.
[135] Winkelman, M. (2003). Complementary therapy for addiction: "Drumming out drugs. " *American Journal of Public Health*, *93*, 647–651.
[136] Carroll, J. F. & McGinley, J. J. (2000). An agency follow-up outcome study of graduates from four inner-city therapeutic community programs. *Journal of Substance Abuse Treatment*, *18*, 103–118.
[137] Wingo, L. K. (2001). Substance abuse in African American women. *Journal of Cultural Diversity*, *8*, 21–25.
[138] Peterson, S., Berkowitz, G., Cart, C. U. & Brindis, C. (2002). Native American women in alcohol and substance abuse treatment. *Journal of Health Care for the Poor and Underserved*, *13*, 360–378.
[139] Hyun, M. S., Kools, S. & Kim, S. A. (2003). A model of recovery from substance abuse and dependence for Korean adolescents. *Journal of Child and Adolescent Psychiatric Nursing*, *16*(1), 25–34.
[140] Bowser, B. P. & Bilal, R. (2001). Drug treatment effectiveness: African-American culture in recovery. *Journal of Psychoactive Drugs*, *33*, 391–402.
[141] Grunbaum, J. A., Tortolero, S., Weller, N. & Gingiss, P. (2000). Cultural, social, and intrapersonal factors associated with substance use among alternative high school students. *Addictive Behaviors*, *25*, 145–151.
[142] Harwood A. (1981). *Ethnicity and medical care*. Cambridge, MA: Harvard University Press.

[143] Kleinman, A., Eisenberg, L. & Good, B. (1978). Culture, illness, and care: Clinical lessons from anthropologic and crosscultural research. *Annals of Internal Medicine*, *88*, 251–258.
[144] Scott, C. K., Dennis, M. L. & Foss, M. A. (2005).
[145] Wingo, L. K. (2001).
[146] Bowser, B. P. & Bilal, R. (2001).
[147] Flores, G. (2000). Culture and the patient-physician relationship: Achieving cultural competency in health care. *The Journal of Pediatrics*, *136*, 14–23.
[148] Ibid.
[149] Sue, D. W., Arrendondo, P. & McDavis, R. J. (1992). Multicultural counseling competencies and standards: A call to the profession. *Journal of Counseling and Development*, *70*, 477–486.
[150] Sue, D. W., Bernier, Y., Durran, A., Feinberg, L., Pedersen, P. B. & Smith, E. J. et al. (1982). Position paper: Cross-cultural counseling competencies. *Counseling Psychologist*, *10*, 45–52.
[151] Sue, D. W., Arrendondo, P. & McDavis, R. J. (1992).
[152] Sue, D. W., Bernier, Y., Durran, A., Feinberg, L. et al. (1982).
[153] Croteau, J. M., Evans, N. J., Lance, T. S. & Talbot, D. M. (2002). A qualitative study of the interplay between privilege and oppression. *Journal of Multicultural Counseling and Development*, *30*(4), 239–258.
[154] Matthews, C. R., Lorah, P. & Fenton, J. (2006). Treatment experiences of gays and lesbians in recovery from addiction: A qualitative inquiry. *Journal of Mental Health Counseling*, *28*(2), 111–132.
[155] Wingo, L. K. (2001).
[156] Hyun, M. S., Kools, S. & Kim, S. A. (2003).
[157] Bowser, B. P. & Bilal, R. (2001).
[158] Anglin, M. D., Hser, Y. I., Grella, C. E., Longshore, D. & Prendergast, M. L. (2001). Drug treatment careers: Conceptual overview and clinical, research, and policy applications. In F. Tims, C. Leukefeld & J. Platt (Eds.), *Relapse and recovery in addictions* (pp. 18–39). New Haven, CT: Yale University Press.
[159] Dennis, M. L., Scott, C. K. & Hristova, L. (2002). The duration and correlates of substance abuse treatment careers among people entering publicly funded treatment in Chicago. *Drug and Alcohol Dependence*, *66*(Suppl. 2), 44.
[160] Hser, Y. I., Anglin, M. D., Grella, C., Longshore, D. & Prendergast, M. L. (1997). Drug treatment careers. A conceptual framework and existing research findings. *Journal of Substance Abuse Treatment*, *14*, 543–558.
[161] Lamb, S., Greenlick, M. R. & McCarty, D. (1998). *Bridging the gap between practice and research: Forging partnerships with community-based drug and alcohol treatment.* Washington, DC: National Academy Press.
[162] Leshner, A. I. (1997). Drug abuse and addiction treatment research. The next generation. *Archives of General Psychiatry*, *54*, 691–694.
[163] McLellan, A. T., Lewis, D. C., O'Brien, C. P. & Kleber, H. D. (2000). Drug dependence, a chronic medical illness: Implications for treatment, insurance, and outcomes evaluation. *JAMA*, *284*, 1689–1695.
[164] Drake, R. E., Wallach, M. A. & McGovern, M. P. (2005).

[165] Rawson, R. A., Obert, J. L., McCann, M. J. & Ling, W. (1991). Psychological approaches for the treatment of cocaine dependence: A neurobehavioral approach. *Journal of Addictive Disorders*, *11*, 97–119.
[166] Drake, R. E., Wallach, M. A. & McGovern, M. P. (2005).
[167] Irving, L. M., Seidner, A. L., Burling, T. A., Pagliarini, R. & Robbins-Sisco, D. (1998). Hope and recovery from substance dependence in homeless veterans. *Journal of Social and Clinical Psychology*, *17*(4), 389–406.
[168] Magura, S., Knight, E. L., Vogel, H. S., Mahmood, D., Laudet, A. B. & Rosenblum, A. (2003). Mediators of effectiveness in dual-focus self-help groups. *American Journal of Drug and Alcohol Abuse*, *29*, 301–322.
[169] Bewley, A. R. (1993). Addiction and meta-recovery: Wellness beyond the limits of Alcoholics Anonymous. *Alcoholism Treatment Quarterly*, *10*(1/2), 1–22.
[170] Whitfield, C. L. (1984). Stress management and spirituality during recovery: A transpersonal approach. Part II: Being. *Alcoholism Treatment Quarterly*, *1*(2).
[171] Whitfield, C. L. (1984). Stress management and spirituality during recovery: A transpersonal approach. Part III: Transforming. *Alcoholism Treatment Quarterly*, *1*(4).
[172] Grof, S. (1987). Spirituality, addiction, and western science. *ReVision*, *10*(2), 18.
[173] Small, J. (1987). Spiritual emergence and addiction: A transpersonal approach to alcoholism and drug abuse counseling. *ReVision*, *10*(2), 23–36.
[174] Sparks, T. (1987). Transpersonal treatment of addictions: Radical return to roots. *ReVision*, *10*(2), 49–64.
[175] McMillen, C., Howard, M. O., Nower, L. & Chung, S. (2001). Positive by-products of the struggle with chemical dependency. *Journal of Substance Abuse Treatment*, *20*, 69–79.
[176] Irving, L. M., Seidner, A. L. & Burling, T. A. et al. (1998).
[177] Magura, S., Knight, E. L. & Vogel, H. S. et al. (2003).
[178] Hewitt, A. (2004). *Post-traumatic growth in substance misuse*. Annegatan, Finland: Nordic Counsel for Alcohol and Drug Research.
[179] Whitfield, C. L. (1984). Stress management and spirituality during recovery: A transpersonal approach. Part I: Becoming. *Alcoholism Treatment Quarterly*, *1*(1).
[180] Hewitt, A. (2004).
[181] Davidson, L., Stayner, D. A., Nickou, C., Styron, T. H., Rowe, M. & Chinman, M. L. (2001). Simply to be let in: Inclusion as a basis for recovery. *Psychiatric Rehabilitation Journal*, *24*, 375–388.
[182] Deegan, P. E. (1996). Recovery as a journey of the heart. *Psychiatric Rehabilitation Journal*, *19*, 91–97.
[183] Fisher, D. (1994). Health care reform based on an empowerment model of recovery by people with psychiatric disabilities. *Hospital and Community Psychology*, *45*(9), 913–915.
[184] Jacobson, N. & Curtis, L. (2000). Recovery as policy in mental health services: Strategies emerging from the states. *Psychiatric Rehabilitation Journal*, *23*(4), 333–341.
[185] Jacobson, N. & Greenley, D. (2001). What is recovery? A conceptual model and explication. *Psychiatric Services*, *52*(4), 482–485.
[186] Mead, S. & Copeland, M. E. (2000). What recovery means to us: Consumers' perspectives. *Community Mental Health Journal*, *36*(3), 315–328.

[187] Smith, M. K. (2000). Recovery from a severe psychiatric disability: Findings of a qualitative study. *Psychiatric Rehabilitation Journal*, *24*(2), 149–159.

[188] Young, S. L. & Ensing, D. S. (1999). Exploring recovery from the perspective of people with psychiatric disabilities. *Psychiatric Rehabilitation Journal*, *22*, 219–231.

[189] Substance Abuse and Mental Health Services Administration. (2006). *Results from the 2005 National Survey on Drug Use and Health: National findings* (NSDUH Series H-30, DHHS Publication No. SMA 06-4194). Rockville, MD: Office of Applied Studies.

[190] Young, S. L. & Ensing, D. S. (1999).

[191] McMillen, C., Howard, M. O. & Nower, L. et al. (2001).

[192] Young, S. L. & Ensing, D. S. (1999).

[193] Institute of Medicine. (2006).

[194] Substance Abuse and Mental Health Services Administration. (2006).

[195] Office of the Surgeon General. (2001). *Mental Health: Culture, race, and ethnicity: A supplement to mental health: A report of the Surgeon General*. Rockville, MD: U. S. Department of Health and Human Services, Public Health Services.

[196] National Institute of Mental Health. (1998). *Bridging science and service: A report by the National Advisory Mental Health Council's Treatment and Services Workgroup*. Bethesda, MD: National Institute of Mental Health.

[197] Wells, K., Miranda, J., Bruce, M. L., Alegria, M. & Wallerstein, N. (2004). Bridging community intervention and mental health services research. *American Journal of Psychiatry*, *161*, 955–963.

[198] Perlick, D. A. (2001). Special section on stigma as a barrier to recovery: Introduction. *Psychiatric Services*, *52*, 1613–1614.

[199] Link, B. G., Struening, E. L., Neese-Todd, S., Asmussen, S. & Phelan, J. C. (2001). Stigma as a barrier to recovery: The consequences of stigma for the self-esteem of people with mental illnesses. *Psychiatric Services*, *52*(12), 1621–1626.

[200] Marks, A. (2002). Jobs elude former drug addicts. *Christian Science Monitor*. Retrieved from http://www.csmonitor.com/2002/0604/p02s02-ussc.html

[201] Curley, B. (2002). Discrimination against people in recovery rampant, advocates say. *Join Together Online*. Retrieved from http://www.jointogether.org/sa/news/features/reader/0,1854,553416,00. html.

[202] Link, B. G., Struening, E. L., Neese-Todd, S. et al. (2001).

[203] Marks, A. (2002).

[204] Curley, B. (2002).

[205] Humphreys, K., Wing, S., McCarty, D., Chappel, J., Gallant, L., Haberle, B. et al. (2004). Self-help organizations for alcohol and drug problems: Toward evidence-based practice and policy. *Journal of Substance Abuse Treatment*, *26*, 151–158.

[206] Brown, S. A., D'Amico, E. J., McCarthy, D. M. & Tapert, S. F. (2001). Four-year outcomes from adolescent alcohol and drug treatment. *Journal of Studies on Alcohol*, *62*, 381–388.

[207] Brown, S. A., Gleghorn, A., Schuckit, M. A., Myers, M. G. & Mott, M. A. (1996). Conduct disorder among adolescent alcohol and drug abusers. *Journal of Studies on Alcohol*, *57*, 314–324.

[208] Catalano, R. F., Hawkins, J. D., Wells, E. A., Miller, J. & Brewer, D. (1991). Evaluation of the effectiveness of adolescent drug abuse treatment, assessment of risks

for relapse, and promising approaches for relapse prevention. *International Journal of the Addictions*, *25*, 1085–1140.

[209] Richter, S. S., Brown, S. A. & Mott, M. A. (1991). The impact of social support and self-esteem on adolescent substance abuse treatment outcome. *Journal of Substance Abuse*, *3*, 371–385.

[210] Shoemaker, R. H. & Sherry, P. (1991). Posttreatment factors influencing outcome of adolescent chemical dependency treatment. *Journal of Adolescent Chemical Dependency*, *2*(1), 89–106.

[211] Solomon, P. (2004). Peer support/peer provided services underlying processes, benefits, and critical ingredients. *Psychiatric Rehabilitation Journal*, *27*, 392–401.

[212] Solomon, P. & Draine, J. (2001). The state of knowledge of the effectiveness of consumer provided services. *Psychiatric Rehabilitation Journal*, *25*, 20–27.

[213] Christensen, A. & Jacobsen, N. S. (1994). Who (or what) can do psychotherapy: The status and challenge of nonprofessional therapies. *Psychological Science*, *5*, 8–14.

[214] Venner, K. L., Matzger, H. & Forcehimes, A. A. et al. (2006).

[215] Humphreys, K., Wing, S., McCarty, D. et al. (2004).

[216] Brown, S. A., D'Amico, E. J., McCarthy, D. M. et al. (2001).

[217] Brown, S. A., Gleghorn, A., Schuckit, M. A. et al. (1996).

[218] Catalano, R. F., Hawkins, J. D., Wells, E. A. et al. (1991).

[219] Richter, S. S., Brown, S. A., Mott, M. A. (1991).

[220] Shoemaker, R. H. & Sherry, P. (1991).

[221] Jason, L. A., Davis, M. I., Ferrari, J. R. & Bishop, P. D. (2001). Oxford House: A review of research and implications for substance abuse recovery and community research. *Journal of Drug Education*, *31*, 1–27.

[222] Humphreys, K., Huebsch, P. D., Finney, J. W. & Moos, R. H. (1999). A comparative evaluation of substance abuse treatment: Substance abuse treatment can enhance the effectiveness of self-help groups. *Alcoholism, Clinical and Experimental Research*, *23*, 558–563.

[223] Venner, K. L., Matzger, H. & Forcehimes, A. A. et al. (2006).

[224] Wingo, L. K. (2001).

[225] Florentine, R. (1999).

[226] Morgenstern, J., Labouvie, E., McCrady et al. (1997).

[227] Jason, L. A., Davis, M. I., Ferrari, J. R. et al. (2001).

[228] Humphreys, K., Huebsch, P. D., Finney, J. W. et al. (1999).

[229] Jason, L. A., Davis, M. I. & Ferrari, J. R. (2007). The need for substance abuse aftercare: Longitudinal analysis of Oxford House. *Addictive Behaviors*, *32*, 803–818.

[230] Mankowski, E. S., Humphreys, K. & Moos, R. H. (2001). Individual and contextual predictors of involvement in twelve-step self-help groups after substance abuse treatment. *American Journal of Community Psychology*, *29*, 537–563.

[231] Timko, C., Moos, R. H., Finney, J. W. & Moos, B. S. (1994). Outcome of treatment for alcohol abuse and involvement in Alcoholics Anonymous among previously untreated problem drinkers. *Journal of Mental Health Administration*, *21*(2), 145–160.

[232] Fiorentine, R. & Hillhouse, M. P. (2000). Exploring the additive effects of drug misuse treatment and twelve-step involvement: Does Twelve-Step ideology matter? *Substance Use and Misuse*, *35*, 367–397.

[233] Emrick, C. D., Tonigan, J. S., Montgomery, H. & Little, L. (1993). Alcoholics Anonymous: What is currently known. In B. S. McCrady & W. R. Miller (Eds.), *Research on Alcoholics Anonymous* (41–76). Brunswick, NJ: Rutgers Center of Alcohol Studies.

[234] Tucker, J. A., Vuchinich, R. E. & Gladsjo, J. A. (1994). Environmental events surrounding natural recovery from alcohol-related problems. *Journal of Studies on Alcohol*, *55*, 401–411.

[235] McKay, J. R., McLellan, A. T., Alterman, A. I., Cacciola, J. S., Rutherford, M. J. & O'Brien, C. P. (1998). Predictors of participation in aftercare sessions and self-help groups following completion of intensive outpatient treatment for substance abuse. *Journal of Studies on Alcohol*, *59*, 152–162.

[236] Fiorentine, R. & Hillhouse, M. (2000). Drug treatment and 12-step participation: The additive effects of integrated recovery activities. *Journal of Substance Abuse Treatment*, *18*(1), 65–74.

[237] Hoffmann, N., Harrison, P. & Belille, C. (1983). Alcoholics Anonymous after treatment: Attendance and abstinence. *International Journal of the Addictions*, *18*(3), 311–318.

[238] Florentine, R. (1999).

[239] Fiorentine, R. & Hillhouse, M. P. (2000).

[240] Emrick, C. D., Tonigan, J. S., Montgomery, H. et al. (1993).

[241] Hoffmann, N., Harrison, P. & Belille, C. (1983).

[242] Cohen, C., Humphreys, K. & Moos, R. H. (1997). Social and community resources and long-term recovery from treated and untreated alcoholism. *Journal of Studies on Alcohol*, *58*(3), 231–238.

[243] Emrick, C. D. (1987). Alcoholics Anonymous: Affiliation processes and effectiveness as treatment. *Alcoholism, Clinical and Experimental Research*, *11*, 416–423.

[244] Kingree, J. B. (1995). Understanding gender differences in psychosocial functioning and treatment retention. *American Journal of Drug and Alcohol Abuse*, *21*(2), 267–281.

[245] McKay, J. R., Alterman, A. I., McLellan, A. T. & Snider, E. C. (1994). Treatment goals, continuity of care, and outcome in a day hospital substance abuse rehabilitation program. *American Journal of Psychiatry*, *151*, 254– 259.

[246] Timko, C. & Sempel, J. M. (2004). Intensity of acute services, self-help attendance and one-year outcomes among dual diagnosis patients. *Journal of Studies on Alcohol*, *65*, 274–282.

[247] Jason, L. A., Davis, M. I., Ferrari, J. R. et al. (2001).

[248] Jason, L. A., Davis, M. I. & Ferrari, J. R. (2007).

[249] Biernacki, P. (1986). *Pathways from heroin addiction: Recovery without treatment.* Philadelphia: Temple University Press.

[250] Gruber, K. J., Fleetwood, T. W. & Herring, M. W. (2001). In-home continuing care services for substance-affected families: The bridges program. *Social Work*, *46*, 267–277.

[251] Miller, W. R. (1998).

[252] Landry, M. J. (1994). *Understanding drugs of abuse: The processes of addiction, treatment, and recovery*. Arlington, VA: American Psychiatric Publishing.

[253] Davis, K. E. & O'Neill, S. J. (2005). A focus group analysis of relapse prevention strategies for persons with substance use and mental disorders. *Psychiatric Services*, *56*, 1288–1291.
[254] Moos, R. H. (1994). Why do some people recover from alcohol dependence, whereas others continue to drink and become worse over time? *Addiction*, *89*, 31–34.
[255] Miller, W. R. & Rollnick, S. (2002).
[256] Cohen, C., Humphreys, K. & Moos, R. H. (1997).
[257] Granfield, R. & Cloud, W. (2001).
[258] Ibid.
[259] Vaillant, G. E. (1988). What can long-term follow-up teach us about relapse and prevention of relapse in addiction? *British Journal of Addictions*, *83*, 1147–1157.
[260] Miller, W. R. (1996).
[261] Landry, M. J. (1994).
[262] Davis, K. E. & O'Neill, S. J. (2005).
[263] Moos, R. H. (1994).
[264] Vaillant, G. E. (1988).
[265] Miller, W. R. & Rollnick, S. (2002).
[266] Flynn, P. M., Joe, G. W., Broome, K. M. et al. (2003).
[267] Margolis, R., Kilpatrick, A. & Mooney, B. (2000). A retrospective look at long-term adolescent recovery: Clinicians talk to researchers. *Journal of Psychoactive Drugs*, *32*, 117–125.
[268] Margolis, R., Kilpatrick, A. & Mooney, B. (2000).
[269] Kessler, R. C. (1994). The National Comorbidity Survey of the United States. *International Review of Psychiatry*, *6*, 365–376.
[270] Dawson, D. A. (1996). Correlates of past-year status among treated and untreated persons with former alcohol dependence: United States, 1992. *Alcoholism, Clinical and Experimental Research*, *20*, 771–779.
[271] Robins, L. N. & Regier, D. A. (1991). *Psychiatric disorders in America: The Epidemiologic Catchment Area Study*. New York: Free Press.
[272] Schutte, K. K., Nichols, K. A., Brennan, P. L. & Moos, R. H. (2003). A ten-year follow-up of older problem drinkers: Risk of relapse and implications of successfully sustained remission. *Journal of Studies on Alcohol*, *64*(3), 367–374.
[273] Ojesjo, L. (1981). Long-term outcome in alcohol abuse alcoholism among males in the Lundby general population, Sweden. *British Journal of Addictions*, *76*, 391–400.
[274] Dawson, D. A., Grant, B. F., Stinson, F. S., Chou, P. S., Huang, B. & Ruan, W. J. (2005). Recovery from DSM-IV alcohol dependence: United States, 2001-2002. *Addiction*, *100*, 281–292.
[275] Vaillant, G. E. (2003). A 60-year follow-up of alcoholic men. *Addiction*, *98*, 1043–1051.
[276] Helzer, J. E., Burnam, A. & McEvoy, L. T. (1991). Alcohol abuse and dependence. In L. N. Robins & D. A. Regier (Eds.), *Psychiatric disorders in America: The Epidemiologic Catchment Area Study* (81–115). New York: Free Press.
[277] Dawson, D. A. (1996).
[278] Faces and Voices of Recovery. (2001). *The road to recovery: A landmark national study on the public perceptions of alcoholism and barriers to treatment*. San Francisco: Peter D. Hart Research Associates/The Recovery Institute.

[279] Brigham, T. (1979). Some effects of choice on academic performance. In L. C. Perlmuter & R. A. Monty (Eds.), *Choice and perceived control*. Hillsdale, NJ: Lawrence Erlbaum.

[280] Laugharne, R. & Priebe, S. (2006). Trust, choice and power in mental health: A literature review. *Social Psychiatry and Psychiatric Epidemiology*, *41*(11), 843–852.

[281] Langer, E. & Rodin, J. (1976). The effects of choice and enhanced personal responsibility for the aged: A field experiment in an institutional setting. *Journal of Personality and Social Psychology*, *34*, 191–198.

[282] Calsyn, R. J., Winter, J. P. & Morse, G. A. (2000). Do consumers who have a choice of treatment have better outcomes? *Community Mental Health Journal*, *36*, 149–160.

[283] Thompson, C. E. & Wankel, L. M. (1980). The effects of perceived activity choice upon frequency of exercise behavior. *Journal of Applied Psychology*, *10*, 436–443.

[284] Rokke, P. D., Tomhave, J. A. & Jocic, Z. (1999). The role of client choice and target selection in self-management therapy for depression in older adults. *Psychology of the Aging*, *14*(1), 155–169.

[285] Kissin, B., Platz, A. & Su, W. H. (1971). Selective factors in treatment choice and outcome in alcoholics. In N. K. Mello and J. K. Mendelson (Eds.), *Recent advances in studies of alcoholism* (NIMH Publication No. [HSM] 71–9045, 781–802). Washington, DC: U. S. Government Printing Office.

[286] Miller, W. R. (1985). Motivation for treatment: A review with special emphasis on alcoholism. *Psychological Bulletin*, *98*, 84–107.

[287] Langer, E. & Rodin, J. (1976).

[288] Calsyn, R. J., Winter, J. P. & Morse, G. A. (2000).

[289] Thompson, C. E. & Wankel, L. M. (1980).

[290] Rokke, P. D., Tomhave, J. A. & Jocic, Z. (1999).

[291] McCrady, B. S., Noel, N. E., Abrams, D. B., Stout, R. L., Nelson, H. F. & Hay, W. M. (1986). Comparative effectiveness of three types of spouse involvement in outpatient behavioral alcoholism treatment. *Journal of Studies on Alcohol*, *47*(6), 459–467.

[292] O'Farrell, T. J., Cutter, H. S. G. & Floyd, F. J. (1985). Evaluating behavioral marital therapy for male alcoholics: Effects on marital adjustment and communication from before to after therapy. *Behavior Therapy*, *16*, 147– 167.

[293] Noel, N. E., McCrady, B. S., Stout, R. L. & Fisher-Nelson, H. (1987). Predictors of attrition from an outpatient alcoholism treatment program for couples. *Journal of Studies on Alcohol*, *48*(3), 229–235.

[294] Higgins, S. T., Budney, A. J., Bickel, W. K. & Badger, G. J. (1994). Participation of significant others in outpatient behavioral treatment predicts greater cocaine abstinence. *The American Journal of Drug and Alcohol Abuse*, *20*, 47–56.

[295] Jason, L. A., Davis, M. I. & Ferrari, J. R. (2007).

[296] McCrady, B. S. (2004). To have but one true friend: Implications for practice of research on alcohol use disorders and social networks. *Psychology of Addictive Behaviors*, *18*, 113–121.

[297] Drake, R. E., Wallach, M. A. & McGovern, M. P. (2005).

[298] Gruber, K. J. & Fleetwood, T. W. (2004). In-home continuing care services for substance use affected families. *Substance Use and Misuse*, *39*, 1379–1403.

[299] Ibid.

[300] Brown, S. & Lewis, V. (1998). *The Alcoholic Family in Recovery. A Developmental Model*. New York: The Guilford Press.

[301] Carten, A. J. (1996). Mothers in recovery: Rebuilding families in the aftermath of addiction. *Social Work*, *41*, 214–223.

[302] Donovan, D. M. (1998). Continuing care: Promoting the maintenance of change. In: W. R. Miller & N. Heather (Eds.), *Treating addictive behaviors* (2nd ed.). New York: Plenum Press.

[303] Higgins, C., Duxbury, L. & Lee, C. (1994). Impact of life-cycle stage and gender on the ability to balance work and family responsibilities. *Family Relations*, *43*(2), 144–150.

[304] O'Farrell, T. J., Choquette, K. A., Cutter, H. S., Brown, E. D. & McCourt, W. F. (1993). Behavioral marital therapy with and without additional couples relapse prevention sessions for alcoholics and their wives. *Journal of Studies on Alcohol*, *54*, 652–666.

[305] Simpson, D. & Joe, G. (2003). A longitudinal evaluation of treatment engagement and recovery stages. *Journal of Substance Abuse Treatment*, *27*, (2), 89-97.

[306] Finney, J. W., Noyes, C. A., Coutts, A. I. & Moos, R. H. (1998). Evaluating substance abuse treatment process models: Changes on proximal outcome variables during 12-step and cognitive-behavioral treatment. *Journal of Studies on Alcohol*, *59*, 371–380.

[307] Granfield, R. & Cloud, W. (2001).

[308] Laudet, A. B., Morgen, K. & White, W. L. (2006).

[309] Weisner, C., Delucchi, K., Matzger, H. & Schmidt, L. (2003). The role of community services and informal support on five-year drinking trajectories of alcohol dependent and problem drinkers. *Journal of Studies on Alcohol*, *64*, 862–873.

[310] Berkman, L. F. (2000). Social support, social networks, social cohesion and health. *Social Work and Health Care*, *31*, 3–14.

[311] Azrin, N. H., Sisson, R. W., Meyers, R. & Godley, M. (1982). Alcoholism treatment by disulfiram and community reinforcement therapy. *Journal of Behavior Therapy and Experimental Psychiatry*, *13*, 105–112.

[312] McCrady, B. S., Noel, N. E., Abrams, D. B. et al. (1986).

[313] O'Farrell, T. J., Cutter, H. S. G. & Floyd, F. J. (1985).

[314] Barber, J. G. & Crisp, B. R. (1995). The "pressures to change"' approach to working with the partners of heavy drinkers. *Addiction*, *90*(2), 269–276.

[315] O'Farrell, T. J., Choquette, K. A., Cutter, H. S. et al. (1993).

[316] Higgins, S. T., Budney, A. J., Bickel, W. K. et al. (1994).

[317] Hser, Y. I., Polinsky, M. L., Maglione, M. & Anglin, M. D. (1999). Matching clients' needs with drug treatment services. *Journal of Substance Abuse Treatment*, *16*, 299–305.

[318] McLellan, A. T., Grissom, G. R., Brill, P., Durell, J., Metzger, D. S. & O'Brien, C. P. (1993). Private substance abuse treatments: Are some programs more effective than others? *Journal of Substance Abuse Treatment*, *10*(3), 243–254.

[319] McLellan, A. T., Alterman, A. I., Metzger, D. S., Grissom, G. R., Woody, G. E., Luborsky, L. et al. (1994). Similarity of outcome predictors across opiate, cocaine, and alcohol treatments: Role of treatment services. *Journal of Consulting and Clinical Psychology*, *62*(6), 1141–1158.

[320] Pringle, J. L., Edmondston, L. A., Holland, C. L., Kirisci, L., Emptage, N., Balavage, V. K. et al. (2002). The role of wrap around services in retention and outcome in

substance abuse treatment: Findings from the Wrap Around Services Impact Study. *Addictive Disorders and their Treatment*, *1*(4), 109–118.

[321] Devine, J. A. & Wright, J. D. (1997). Losing the housing game. The leveling effects of substance abuse. *American Journal of Orthopsychiatry*, *67*, 618–631.

[322] Brecht, M. L., Anglin, M. D. & Wang, J. C. (1993). Treatment effectiveness for legally coerced versus voluntary methadone maintenance clients. *American Journal of Drug and Alcohol Abuse*, *19*, 89–106.

[323] DeLeon, G. (1988). Legal pressure in therapeutic communities. *Journal of Drug Issues*, *18*, 625–640.

[324] Hser, Y. I., Polinsky, M. L., Maglione, M. et al. (1999).

[325] Pringle, J. L., Edmondston, L. A., Holland, C. L. et al. (2002).

[326] Friedmann, P. D., Hendrickson, J. C., Gerstein, D. R. & Zhang, Z. (2004). Designated case managers as facilitators of medical and psychosocial service delivery in addiction treatment programs. *Journal of Behavior Health Services Research*, *31*, 86–97.

[327] Hser, Y. I., Polinsky, M. L., Maglione, M. et al. (1999).

[328] McLellan, A. T., Grissom, G. R., Brill, P. et al. (1993).

[329] Pringle, J. L., Edmondston, L. A., Holland, C. L. et al. (2002).

[330] Friedmann, P. D., Hendrickson, J. C., Gerstein, D. R. et al. (2004).

[331] Kessler, R. C., Berglund, P., Demler, O., Jin, R., Merikangas, K. R. & Walters, E. E. (2005). Lifetime prevalence and age-of-onset distributions of DSM-IV disorders in the National Comorbidity Survey Replication. *Archives of General Psychiatry*, *62*, 593–602.

[332] Ross, H. E., Glaser, F. B. & Germanson, T. (1988). The prevalence of psychiatric disorders in patients with alcohol and other drug problems. *Archives of General Psychiatry*, *45*, 1023–1031.

[333] Anglin, M. D., Hser, Y. I. & Booth, M. W. (1987). Sex differences in addict careers. 4. Treatment. *American Journal of Drug and Alcohol Abuse*, *13*, 253–280.

[334] Grella, C. E. & Joshi, V. (1999). Gender differences in drug treatment careers among clients in the National Drug Abuse Treatment Outcome Study. *American Journal of Drug and Alcohol Abuse*, *25*(3), 385–406.

[335] Wechsberg, W. M., Craddock, S. G. & Hubbard, R. L. (1998). How are women who enter substance abuse treatment different than men? A gender comparison from the Drug Abuse Treatment Outcome Study (DATOS). *Drugs and Society*, *13*(1/2), 97–115.

[336] Tims, F., Leukefeld, C. & Platt, J. (2001). *Relapse and recovery in addictions*. New Haven, CT: Yale University Press.

[337] Halfon, N. & Hochstein, M. (2002). Life course health development: An integrated framework for developing health, policy, and research. *Milbank Quarterly*, *80*, 433–79, iii.

[338] Antonucci, T. C. (1990). Social supports and social relationships. In R. H. Binstock (Ed.), *Handbook of aging and the social sciences* (3rd ed.). New York:Van Nostrand Reinhold.

[339] Rice, C., Longabaugh, R., Beattie, M. & Noel, N. (1993). Age group differences in response to treatment for problematic alcohol use. *Addiction*, *88*(10), 1369–1375.

[340] Bartels, S. J., Blow, F. C., Brockmann, L. M. & Van Citters, A. D. (2005). *Substance abuse and mental health among older Americans: The state of the knowledge and future directions.* Rockville, MD: Westat.

[341] Blow, F. C., Walton, M. A., Chermack, S. T., Mudd, S. A. & Brower, K. J. (2000). Older adult treatment outcome following elder-specific inpatient alcoholism treatment. *Journal of Substance Abuse Treatment*, *19*(1), 67–75.
[342] Schonfeld, L. & Dupree, L. W. (1995). Treatment approaches for older problem drinkers. *International Journal of the Addictions*, *30*(13–14), 1819–1842.
[343] Benshoff, J. J., Harrawood, L. K. & Koch, D. S. (2003). Substance abuse and the elderly: Unique issues and concerns. *Journal of Rehabilitation*, *69*, 43–48.
[344] Satre, D. D., Mertens, J. R., Arean, P. A. & Weisner, C. (2004). Five-year alcohol and drug treatment outcomes of older adults versus middle-aged and younger adults in a managed care program. *Addiction*, *99*, 1286–1297.
[345] Tims, F., Leukefeld, C. & Platt, J. (2001).
[346] Blow, F. C., Walton, M. A., Chermack, S. T. et al. (2000).
[347] Schonfeld, L. & Dupree, L. W. (1995).
[348] Benshoff, J. J., Harrawood, L. K. & Koch, D. S. (2003).
[349] Berk, L. E. (2007). *Development through the lifespan* (4th ed.). Boston: Allyn & Bacon.
[350] Featherman, D. L. & Lerner, R. M. (1985). Ontogenesis and sociogenesis: Problematics for theory and research about development and socialization across the lifespan. *American Sociological Review*, *50*(5), 659– 676.
[351] Rice, C., Longabaugh, R., Beattie, M. et al. (1993).
[352] Schonfeld, L. & Dupree, L. W. (1995).
[353] Bartels, S. J., Blow, F. C., Brockmann, L. M. et al. (2005).
[354] Blow, F. C., Walton, M. A., Chermack, S. T. et al. (2000).
[355] Fortney, J. C., Booth, B. M., Blow, F. C. & Bunn, J. Y. (1995). The effects of travel barriers and age on the utilization of alcoholism treatment aftercare. *American Journal of Drug and Alcohol Abuse*, *21*, 391–406.
[356] Rice, C., Longabaugh, R., Beattie, M. et al. (1993).
[357] Bartels, S. J., Blow, F. C., Brockmann, L. M. et al. (2005).
[358] Blow, F. C., Walton, M. A., Chermack, S. T. et al. (2000).
[359] Schonfeld, L. & Dupree, L. W. (1995).
[360] Fillmore, K. M., Grant, M., Hartka, E. et al. (1988).
[361] Sobell, L. C., Ellingstad, T. P. & Sobell, M. B. (2000).
[362] Humphreys, K., Moos, R. H. & Finney, J. W. (1995). Two pathways out of drinking problems without professional treatment. *Addictive Behaviors*, *20*, 427–441.
[363] Granfield, R. & Cloud, W. (2001).
[364] Drake, R. E., Wallach, M. A. & McGovern, M. P. (2005).
[365] Hser, Y. I., Grella, C. E., Hsieh, S. C., Anglin, M. D. & Brown, B. S. (1999). Prior treatment experience related to process and outcomes in DATOS. *Drug and Alcohol Dependence*, *57*, 137–150.
[366] Simpson, D. D., Joe, G. W., Greener, J. M. & Rowan-Szal, G. A. (2000). Modeling year 1 outcomes with treatment process and post-treatment social influences. *Substance Use and Misuse*, *35*, 1911–1930.
[367] Broome, K. M., Simpson, D. D. & Joe, G. W. (2002). The role of social support following short-term inpatient treatment. *American Journal of Addictions*, *11*, 57–65.
[368] Bradizza, C. M. & Stasiewicz, P. R. (2003). Qualitative analysis of high-risk drug and alcohol use situations among severely mentally ill substance abusers. *Addictive Behaviors*, *28*, 157–169.

[369] Bradizza, C. M., Stasiewicz, P. R. & Carey, K. B. (1998). High-risk alcohol and drug use situations among seriously mentally ill inpatients: A preliminary investigation. *Addictive Behaviors*, *23*, 555–560.
[370] Alverson, H., Alverson, M. & Drake, R. E. (2000). An ethnographic study of the longitudinal course of substance abuse among people with severe mental illness. *Community Mental Health Journal*, *36*, 557–569.
[371] Sells, D. J., Rowe, M., Fisk, D. & Davidson, L. (2003). Violent victimization of persons with co-occurring psychiatric and substance use disorders. *Psychiatric Services*, *54*, 1253–1257.
[372] Sells, D. J., Rowe, M., Fisk, D. et al. (2003).
[373] Kisthardt, W. (1997). The strengths model of case management: Principles and helping functions. In D. Saleeby (Ed.), *The Strengths Perspective in Social Work Practice* (2nd ed., 97–114). New York: Longman.
[374] Rapp, C. A. (1998). *The strengths model: Case management with people suffering from severe and persistent mental illness*. New York: Oxford University Press.
[375] Carten, A. J. (1996).
[376] Rapp, C. A. (1998).
[377] Blankertz, L., McKay, C. & Robinson, S. (1998). Work as a rehabilitative tool for individuals with dual diagnosis. *Journal of Vocational Rehabilitation*, *11*, 113–123.
[378] Comerford, A. W. (1999). Work dysfunction and addiction: Common roots. *Journal of Substance Abuse Treatment*, *16*, 247–253.
[379] Dickinson, K. & Maynard, R. (1981). *The impact of supported work on ex-addicts*. New York: MDRC.
[380] Platt, J. J. (1995). Vocational rehabilitation of drug abusers. *Psychological Bulletin*, *117*, 416–433.
[381] Room, R. (1998). Drinking patterns and alcohol-related social problems: Frameworks for analysis in developing societies. *Drug and Alcohol Review*, *17*, 389–398.
[382] Pringle, J. L., Edmondston, L. A., Holland, C. L. et al. (2002).
[383] McDaid, D. & Thornicroft, G. (2005). *Mental health II: Balancing institutional and community-based care*. World Health Organization Regional Office for Europe.
[384] Trieman, N., Leff, J. & Glover, G. (1999). Outcome of long stay psychiatric patients resettled in the community: Prospective cohort study. *British Medical Journal*, *319*, 13–16.
[385] Ibid.
[386] Harrison, L. D. (2001). The revolving prison door for drug involved offenders: Challenges and opportunities. *Crime & Delinquency*, *47*(3), 462–485.
[387] Knight, K., Simpson, D. D. & Hiller, M. (1999). Three-year reincarceration outcomes for in-prison therapeutic community treatment in Texas. *Prison Journal*, *79*, 337–351.
[388] Haggerty, J. L., Reid, R. J., Freeman, G. K., Starfield, B. H., Adair, C. E. & McKendry, R. (2003). Continuity of care: A multidisciplinary review. *British Medical Journal*, *327*, 1219–1221.
[389] Ibid.
[390] Moos, R. H. (2003). Addictive disorders in context: Principles and puzzles of effective treatment and recovery. *Psychology of Addictive Behaviors*, *17*, 3–12.
[391] Miller, W. R. & Hester, R. K. (1986). Inpatient alcoholism treatment: Who benefits? *American Psychologist*, *41*, 794–805.

[392] Fortney, J. C., Booth, B. M., Blow, F. C. et al. (1995).

[393] McKay, J. R. (2001). Effectiveness of continuing care interventions for substance abusers: Implications for study of long-term treatment effects. *Evaluation Review*, *25*(2), 211–232.

[394] Gruber, K. J., Fleetwood, T. W. & Herring, M. W. (2001).

[395] Gruber, K. J. & Fleetwood, T. W. (2004).

[396] Godley, M. D., Godley, S. H., Dennis, M. L., Funk, R. & Passetti, L. L. (2002). Preliminary outcomes from the assertive continuing care experiment for adolescents discharged from residential treatment. *Journal of Substance Abuse Treatment*, *23*, 21–32.

[397] Dennis, M., Scott, C. K. & Funk, R. (2003). An experimental evaluation of recovery management checkups (RMC) for people with chronic substance use disorders. *Evaluation and Program Planning*, *26*, 339–352.

[398] Donovan, D. M. (1998).

[399] Godley, M. D., Godley, S. H., Dennis, M., Funk, R. & Passetti, L. L. (2007). The effect of assertive continuing care on continuing care linkage, adherence and abstinence following residential treatment for adolescents with substance use disorders. *Addiction*, *102*, 81–93.

[400] Godley, M. D., Godley, S. H., Dennis, M. et al. (2007).

[401] Druss, B. G. & von Esenwein, S. A. (2006). Improving general medical care for persons with mental and addictive disorders: Systematic review. *General Hospital Psychiatry*, *28*, 145–153.

[402] Rothman, J., Rudnick, D., Slifer, M., Agins, B., Heiner, K. & Birkhead, G. (2007). Co-located substance use treatment and HIV prevention and primary care services, New York State, 1990-2002: A model for effective service delivery to a high-risk population. *Journal of Urban Health*, *84*, 226–242.

[403] Hitchcock, H. C., Stainback, R. D. & Roque, G. M. (1995). Effects of halfway house placement on retention of patients in substance abuse aftercare. *American Journal of Drug and Alcohol Abuse*, *21*, 379–390.

[404] Rosenheck, R. & Gallup, P. (1991). Involvement in an outreach and residential treatment program for homeless mentally ill veterans. *Journal of Nervous and Mental Disease*, *179*, 750–754.

[405] Moos, R. H., Finney, J. W., Ouimette, P. C. & Suchinsky, R. T. (1999). A comparative evaluation of substance abuse treatment: I. Treatment orientation, amount of care, and 1-year outcomes. *Alcoholism, Clinical and Experimental Research*, *23*, 529–536.

[406] Farabee, D., Prendergast, M. Cartier, J., Wexler, H., Knight, K. & Anglin, M. D. (1999). Barriers to implementing effective correctional drug treatment programs. *Prison Journal*, *7*(2), 150–162.

[407] Wolff, N., Plemmons, D., Veysey, B. & Brandli, A. (2002). Release planning for inmates with mental illness compared with those who have other chronic illnesses. *Psychiatric Services*, *53*, 1469–1471.

[408] Sung, H. E. & Richter, L. (2006). Contextual barriers to successful reentry of recovering drug offenders. *Journal of Substance Abuse Treatment*, *31*, 365–374.

[409] Butzin, C. A., Martin, S. S. & Inciardi, J. A. (2002). Evaluating component effects of a prison-based treatment continuum. *Journal of Substance Abuse Treatment*, *22*, 63–69.

[410] Wexler, H. K., Melnick, G., Lowe, L. & Peters, J. (1999). Three-year reincarceration outcomes for Amity in-prison therapeutic community and aftercare in California. *Prison Journal*, *79*, 321–336.

[411] Broome, K. M., Simpson, D. D. & Joe, G. W. (1999). Patient and program attributes related to treatment process indicators in DATOS. *Drug and Alcohol Dependence*, *57*, 127–135.

[412] Joe, G. W., Simpson, D. D., Dansereau, D. F. & Rowan-Szal, G. A. (2001). Relationships between counseling rapport and drug abuse treatment outcomes. *Psychiatric Services*, *52*, 1223–1229.

[413] Alverson, H., Alverson, M. & Drake, R. E. (2001). Social patterns of substance use among people with dual diagnoses. *Mental Health Services Research*, *3*, 3–14.

[414] Moos, R. H., Finney, J. W., Ouimette, P. C., et al. (1999).

[415] Farabee, D., Prendergast, M., Cartier, J., et al. (1999).

[416] Wolff, N., Plemmons, D., Veysey, B. et al. (2002).

[417] Sung, H. E. & Richter, L. (2006).

[418] Butzin, C. A., Martin, S. S. & Inciardi, J. A. (2002).

[419] Wexler, H. K., Melnick, G., Lowe, L. et al. (1999).

[420] Broome, K. M., Simpson, D. D. & Joe, G. W. (1999).

[421] Ibid.

[422] Joe, G. W., Simpson, D. D., Dansereau, D. F. et. al. (2001).

[423] Alverson, H., Alverson, M. & Drake, R. E. (2001).

[424] Green, J. M. (1996). Engagement and empathy: A pilot study of the therapeutic alliance in outpatient child psychiatry. *Child Psychology and Psychiatry Review*, *1*, 130–138.

[425] Meier, P. S., Barrowclough, C. & Donmall, M. C. (2005). The role of the therapeutic alliance in the treatment of substance misuse: A critical review of the literature. *Addiction*, *100*, 304–316.

[426] Felton, B. J., Barr, A., Clark, G. & Tsemberis, S. J. (2006). ACT team members' responses to training in recovery-oriented practices. *Psychiatric Rehabilitation Journal*, *30*, 112–119.

[427] Lorig, K. R. & Holman, H. (2003).

[428] Ibid, 2.

[429] Ibid, 1.

[430] Moos, R. H. (2003).

[431] Simpson, D. D. (2004). A conceptual framework for drug treatment process and outcomes. *Journal of Substance Abuse Treatment*, *27*, 99–121.

[432] Connors, G. J., Carroll, K. M., DiClemente, C. C., Longabaugh, R. & Donovan, D. M. (1997). The therapeutic alliance and its relationship to alcoholism treatment participation and outcome. *Journal of Consulting and Clinical Psychology*, *65*, 588–598.

[433] Dearing, R. L., Barrick, C., Dermen, K. H. & Walitzer, K. S. (2005). Indicators of client engagement: Influences on alcohol treatment satisfaction and outcomes. *Psychology of Addictive Behaviors*, *19*, 71–78.

[434] Miller, W. R. & Wilbourne, P. L. (2002). Mesa Grande: A methodological analysis of clinical trials of treatments for alcohol use disorders. *Addiction*, *97*, 265–277.

[435] Dearing, R. L., Barrick, C., Dermen, K. H., et al. (2005).

[436] Belding, M. A., Iguchi, M. Y., Morral, A. R. & McLellan, A. T. (1997). Assessing the helping alliance and its impact in the treatment of opiate dependence. *Drug and Alcohol Dependence*, *48*, 51–59.

[437] Petry, N. M. & Bickel, W. K. (1999). Therapeutic alliance and psychiatric severity as predictors of completion of treatment for opioid dependence. *Psychiatric Services*, *50*, 219–227.

[438] Diamond, G. M., Diamond, G. S. & Liddle, H. A. (2000). The therapist-parent alliance in family-based therapy for adolescents. *Journal of Clinical Psychology*, *56*, 1037–1050.

[439] Kasarabada, N. D., Hser, Y. I., Boles, S. M. & Huang, Y. C. (2002). Do patients' perceptions of their counselors influence outcomes of drug treatment? *Journal of Substance Abuse Treatment*, *23*(4), 327–334.

[440] Ilgen, M., Tiet, Q., Finney, J. & Moos, R. H. (2006). Self-efficacy, therapeutic alliance, and alcohol-use disorder treatment outcomes. *Journal of Studies on Alcohol*, *67*(3), 465–472.

[441] Ilgen, M. A., McKellar, J., Moos, R. & Finney, J. W. (2006). Therapeutic alliance and the relationship between motivation and treatment outcomes in patients with alcohol use disorder. *Journal of Substance Abuse Treatment*, *31*(2), 157–162. Epub 2006 Jul 13.

[442] Carten, A. J. (1996).

[443] Siegal, H. A., Fisher, J. H., Rapp, R. C., Kelliher, C. W., Wagner, J. H., O'Brien, W. F., et al. (1996). Enhancing substance abuse treatment with case management: Its impact on employment. *Journal of Substance Abuse Treatment*, *13*(2), 93–98.

[444] Hall, J. A., Carswell, C., Walsh, E., Huber, D. L. & Jampoler, J. S. (2002). Iowa case management: Innovative social casework. *Social Work*, *47*, 132–141.

[445] Rapp, R. C., Kelliher, C. W., Fisher, J. H. & Hall, F. J. (1994). Strengths-based case management. A role in addressing denial in substance abuse treatment. *Journal of Case Management*, *3*, 139–144.

[446] Saleebey, D. (1996). The strengths perspective in social work practice: Extensions and cautions. *Social Work*, *41*, 296–305.

[447] Weick, A., Rapp, C., Sullivan, W. P. & Kisthardt, W. (1989). A strengths perspective for social work practice. *Social Work*, *34* (4): 350–354.

[448] Siegal, H. A., Fisher, J. H., Rapp, R. C. et al. (1996).

[449] Siegal, H. A., Li, L. & Rapp, R. C. (2002). Case management as a therapeutic enhancement: Impact on post-treatment criminality. *Journal of Addictive Disorders*, *21*(4), 37–46.

[450] Rapp, R. C., Siegal, H. A., Li, L. & Saha, P. (1998). Predicting post primary treatment services and drug use outcome: A multivariate analysis. *American Journal of Drug and Alcohol Abuse*, *24*, 603–615.

[451] Arredondo, P., Toperek, R., Brown, S. P., Jones, J., Locke, D. C., Sanchez, J. et al. (1996). Operationalization of the multicultural counseling competencies. *Journal of Multicultural Counseling and Development*, *24*, 42– 78.

[452] Office of Minority Health (2001). *National standards for culturally and linguistically appropriate services in health care: Final report*. Rockville, MD: U. S. Department of Health and Human Services. Retrieved April 2, 2007, from http://www.omhrc.gov/templates/browse. aspx?lvl=2&lvlID=15.

[453] Brach, C. & Fraser, I. (2000). Can cultural competency reduce racial and ethnic health disparities? A review and conceptual model. *Medical Care Research Review, 57* (S1), 181–217.

[454] Lavizzo-Mourey, R. & Mackenzie. E. R. (1996). Cultural competence: Essential measurements of quality for managed care organizations. *Annals of Internal Medicine, 124* (10), 919–920.

[455] Lawson, W. B. (1996). The art and science of the psychopharmacotherapy of African Americans. *Mount Sinai Journal of Medicine, 63*(5–6), 301–305.

[456] Moffic, H. S. & Kinzie, J. D. (1996). The history and future of cross-cultural psychiatric services. *Community Mental Health Journal, 32*(6), 581–592.

[457] Cheung, F. K. & Snowden, L. R. (1990). Community mental health and ethnic minority populations. *Community Mental Health Journal, 26*, 277–291.

[458] Simpson, D. D. (2004).

[459] Office of Minority Health (2001).

[460] Brach, C. & Fraser, I. (2000).

[461] Ford, E. S. & Cooper, R. S. (1995). Implications of race/ethnicity for health and health care use. *Health Services Research, 30*(1), 237–252.

[462] Gornick, M. E., Eggers, P. W., Reilly, T. W., Mentnech, R. M., Fitterman, L. K., Kucken, L. E. et al. (1996). Effects of race and income on mortality and use of services among Medicare beneficiaries. *New England Journal of Medicine, 335*(11), 791–799.

[463] Mayberry, R. M., Mili, F., Vaid, I. G. M., Samadi, A., Ofili, E., McNeal, M. S. et al. (1999). *Racial and ethnic differences in access to medical care: A synthesis of the literature.* Menlo Park, CA: Henry J. Kaiser Family Foundation.

[464] Kington, R. S. & Smith, J. P. (1997). Socioeconomic status and racial and ethnic differences in functional status associated with chronic diseases. *American Journal of Public Health, 87*(5), 805–810.

[465] Williams, D. R. (1999). Race, socioeconomic status, and health: The added effects of racism and discrimination. *Annals of the New York Academy of Sciences, 896*, 173–188.

[466] Nickens, H. W. (1995). The role of race/ethnicity and social class in minority health status. *Health Services Research, 30* (1, Part II), 151–162.

[467] Hyun, M. S., Kools, S. & Kim, S. A. (2003).

[468] Uziel-Miller, N. D., Lyons, J. S., Kissiel, C. & Love, S. (1998). Treatment needs and initial outcomes of a residential recovery program for African-American women and their children. *American Journal of Addictions, 7*, 43–50.

[469] Campbell, C. I. & Alexander, J. A. (2002). Culturally competent treatment practices and ancillary service use in outpatient substance abuse treatment. *Journal of Substance Abuse Treatment, 22*(3), 109–119.

[470] Longshore, D., Grills, C. & Annon, K. (1999). Effects of a culturally congruent intervention on cognitive factors related to drug-use recovery. *Substance Use and Misuse, 34*(9), 1223–1241.

[471] Campbell, C. I. & Alexander, J. A. (2002).

[472] Ehrmin, J. T. (2005). Dimensions of culture care for substance-dependent African American women. *Journal of Transcultural Nursing, 16*, 117–125.

[473] Miller, W. R. (1998).

[474] Miller, W. R., Meyers, R. J. & Hiller-Sturmhofel, S. (1999). The community-reinforcement approach. *Alcohol Research and Health, 23*, 116–121.

[475] Ehrmin, J. T. (2005).
[476] Arnold, R., Avants, S. K., Margolin, A. & Marcotte, D. (2002). Patient attitudes concerning the inclusion of spirituality into addiction treatment. *Journal of Substance Abuse Treatment*, *23*, 319–326.
[477] Avants, S. K., Warburton, L. A. & Margolin, A. (2001). Spiritual and religious support in recovery from addiction among HIV-positive injection drug users. *Journal of Psychoactive Drugs*, *33*, 39–45.
[478] Brizer, D. A. (1993). Religiosity and drug abuse among psychiatric inpatients. *American Journal of Drug and Alcohol Abuse*, *19*, 337–345.
[479] Gorsuch, R. L. (1994). Toward motivational theories of intrinsic religious commitment. *Journal of Science and Studies in Religion*, 33(4), 315–325.
[480] Kendler, K. S., Gardner, C. O. & Prescott, C. A. (1997). Religion, psychopathology, and substance use and abuse: A multimeasure, genetic-epidemiologic study. *American Journal of Psychiatry*, *154*, 322–329.
[481] Mathew, R. J., Georgi, J., Wilson, W. H. & Mathew, V. G. (1996). A retrospective study of the concept of spirituality as understood by recovering individuals. *Journal of Substance Abuse Treatment*, *13*, 67–73.
[482] Miller, W. R. (1998).
[483] Avants, S. K., Warburton, L. A. & Margolin, A. (2001).
[484] Muffler, J., Langrod, J. G. & Larson, D. (1992). "There is a balm in Gilead." Religion and substance abuse treatment. In J. H. Lowinson, P. Ruiz & R. B. Millman (Eds.), *Substance abuse: A comprehensive textbook* (2nd ed., 584–595). Baltimore: Williams & Wilkins.
[485] Laudet, A. B., Morgen, K. & White, W. L. (2006).
[486] Ibid.
[487] Pardini, D. A., Plante, T. G., Sherman, A. & Stump, J. E. (2000). Religious faith and spirituality in substance abuse recovery: Determining the mental health benefits. *Journal of Substance Abuse Treatment*, *19*, 347– 354.
[488] Kondo, C., Iimuro, T., Iwai, K., Kurata, K., Kouda, M., Tachikawa, H. et al. (2000). [A study of recovery factor about drug addiction recovery center (DARC)]. *Nihon Arukoru Yakubutsu Igakkai Zasshi*, *35*, 258–270.
[489] Flynn, P. M., Joe, G. W., Broome, K. M. et al. (2003).
[490] Laudet, A. B., Morgen, K. & White, W. L. (2006). 15.
[491] Ibid.
[492] Miller, W. R. (1998). Why do people change addictive behavior? The 1996 H. David Archibald Lecture. *Addiction*, *93*, 163–172.
[493] Arnold, R., Avants, S. K., Margolin, A. et al. (2002).
[494] Institute of Medicine. (2006).
[495] Humphreys, K., Wing, S., McCarty, D. et al. (2004).
[496] Galanter, M., Dermatis, H., Egelko, S. & De Leon, G. (1998). Homelessness and mental illness in a professional-and peer-led cocaine treatment clinic. *Psychiatric Services*, *49*(4), 533–535.
[497] Bandura, A. (1997). The anatomy of stages of change. *American Journal of Health Promotion*, *12*, 8–10.
[498] Lorig, K. R., Ritter, P., Stewart, A. L. et al. (2001).
[499] Institute of Medicine. (2006).

[500] Bodenheimer, T., Lorig, K., Holman, H. & Grumbach, K. (2002). Patient self-management of chronic disease in primary care. *JAMA*, *288*, 2469–2475.
[501] Moos, R. H., Moos, B. S. & Timko, C. (2006). Gender, Treatment, and Self-Help in Remission from Alcohol Use and Disorders. *Clinical Medical Research*, *4*, 163-174.
[502] Morgenstern, J., Labouvie, E., McCrady, B. S. et al. (1997).
[503] Humphreys, K. (2004). A few apologies, but no regrets. *Addiction*, *99*, 155–156.
[504] Humphreys, K., Mankowski, E., Moos, R. & Finney, J. (1999). Do enhanced friendship networks and active coping mediate the effect of self-help groups on substance abuse? *Annals of Behavioral Medicine*, *21*(1), 54– 60.
[505] McKellar, J., Stewart, E. & Humphreys, K. (2003). Alcoholics anonymous involvement and positive alcohol-related outcomes: Cause, consequence, or just a correlate? A prospective 2-year study of 2,319 alcohol-dependent men. *Journal of Consulting and Clinical Psychology*, *71*, 302–308.
[506] Connors, G. J., Tonigan, J. S. & Miller, W. R. (2001). A longitudinal model of intake symptomatology, AA participation and outcome: Retrospective study of the project MATCH outpatient and aftercare samples. *Journal of Studies on Alcohol*, *62*, 817–825.
[507] Owen, P. L., Slaymaker, V., Tonigan, J. S., McCrady, B. S., Epstein, E. E., Kaskutas, L. A. et al. (2003). Participation in Alcoholics Anonymous: Intended and unintended change mechanisms. *Alcoholism*, *Clinical and Experimental Research*, *27*, 524–532.
[508] Humphreys, K. & Moos, R. (2001). Can encouraging substance abuse patients to participate in self-help groups reduce demand for health care? A quasi-experimental study. *Alcoholism*, *Clinical and Experimental Research*, *25*, 711–716.
[509] Hawkins, J. D. & Catalano, R. F. (1985). Aftercare in drug abuse treatment. *International Journal of the Addictions*, *20*, 917–945.
[510] Johnson, N. P. & Chappel, J. N. (1994). Using AA and other 12-step programs more effectively. *Journal of Substance Abuse Treatment*, *11*(2), 137–142.
[511] Khantzian, E. J. & Mack, J. E. (1994). How AA works and why it's important for clinicians to understand. *Journal of Substance Abuse Treatment*, *11*(2), 77–92.
[512] Connors, G. J., Tonigan, J. S. & Miller, W. R. (2001).
[513] Humphreys, K., Mankowski, E., Moos, R. et al. (1999).
[514] Owen, P. L., Slaymaker, V., Tonigan, J. S. et al. (2003).
[515] Humphreys, K. & Moos, R. (2001).
[516] Johnson, N. P. & Chappel, J. N. (1994).
[517] Khantzian, E. J. & Mack, J. E. (1994).
[518] Hawkins, J. D. & Catalano, R. F. (1985).
[519] Troyer, T. N., Acampora, A. P., O'Connor, L. E. & Berry, J. W. (1995). The changing relationship between therapeutic communities and 12-Step programs: A survey. *Journal of Psychoactive Drugs*, *27*, 177–180.
[520] Fiorentine, R. & Hillhouse, M. P. (2000).
[521] Caldwell, P. E. & Cutter, H. S. (1998). Alcoholics Anonymous affiliation during early recovery. *Journal of Substance Abuse Treatment*, *15*, 221–228.
[522] Etheridge, R. M., Craddock, S. G., Hubbard, R. L. & Rounds-Bryant, J. L. (1999). The relationship of counseling and self-help participation to patient outcomes in DATOS. *Drug and Alcohol Dependence*, *57*, 99– 112.
[523] Vanicelli, M. (1978). Impact of aftercare in the treatment of alcoholics: A cross-lagged panel analysis. *Journal of Studies on Alcohol*, *39*, 1875–1886.

[524] Kissina, W., McLeoda, C. & McKay, J. (2003). The longitudinal relationship between self-help group attendance and course of recovery. *Evaluation and Program Planning*, *26*, 311–323.
[525] Morgenstern, J., Labouvie, E., McCrady, B. S. et al. (1997).
[526] Humphreys, K., Mankowski, E., Moos, R. et al. (1999).
[527] Galanter, M., Egelko, S. & Edwards, H. (1993). Rational recovery: Alternative to AA for addiction? *American Journal of Drug and Alcohol Abuse*, *19*, 499–510.
[528] Brooks, A. J. & Penn, P. E. (2003). Comparing treatments for dual diagnosis: Twelve-step and self-management and recovery training. *American Journal of Drug and Alcohol Abuse*, *29*, 359–383.
[529] Scutchfield, F. D., Ireson, C. & Hall, L. (2004). The voice of the public in public health policy and planning: The role of public judgment. *Journal of Public Health Policy*, *25*, 197–205.
[530] Merzel, C. & D'Afflitti, J. (2003). Reconsidering community-based health promotion: Promise, performance, and potential. *American Journal of Public Health*, *93*(4), 557–574.
[531] Ibid.
[532] Jeffs, L., Law, M., Baker, G. R. & Norton, P. G. (2005). *Patient safety research in Australia, United Kingdom, United States and Canada: A summary of research priority areas, agenda-setting processes, and directions for future research in the context of their patient safety initiatives*. Canadian Patient Safety Institute.
[533] Ibid.
[534] Dwyer, J. (1989). The politics of participation. *Community Health Studies*, *13*, 59–65.
[535] Sofaer, S. (1999). Challenges for the public in negotiating the health system in the 21st century. *Journal of Urban Health*, *76*, 211–228.
[536] Walsh, D. (1996). A journey toward recovery: From the inside out. *Psychiatric Rehabilitation Journal*, *20*(2), 85–90.
[537] Sofaer, S. (1999).
[538] Ibid.
[539] Moggi, F., Hirsbrunner, H. P., Brodbeck, J. & Bachmann, K. M. (1999). One-year outcome of an integrative inpatient treatment for dual diagnosis patients. *Addictive Behaviors*, *24*(4), 589–592.
[540] Weisner, C., Mertens, J., Parthasarathy, S., Moore, C. & Lu, Y. (2001). Integrating primary medical care with addiction treatment: A randomized controlled trial. *JAMA*, *286*, 1715–1723.
[541] Parthasarathy, S., Mertens, J., Moore, C. & Weisner, C. (2003). Utilization and cost impact of integrating substance abuse treatment and primary care. *Medical Care*, *41*, 357–367.
[542] McAlpine, C., Marshall, C. C. & Doran, N. H. (2001). Combining child welfare and substance abuse services: A blended model of intervention. *Child Welfare*, *80*, 129–149.
[543] Friedmann, P. D., Hendrickson, J. C., Gerstein, D. R. et al. (2004).
[544] Weisner, C., Mertens, J., Parthasarathy, S. et al. (2001).
[545] Friedmann, P. D., Lemon, S. C., Stein, M. D., Etheridge, R. M. & D'Aunno, T. A. (2001). Linkage to medical services in the Drug Abuse Treatment Outcome Study. *Medical Care*, *39*, 284–295.

[546] Parthasarathy, S., Mertens, J., Moore, C. et al. (2003).
[547] McAlpine, C., Marshall, C. C. & Doran, N. H. (2001)
[548] McLellan, A. T., Hagan, T. A., Levine, M., Gould, F., Meyers, K., Bencivengo, M. et al. (1998). Supplemental social services improve outcomes in public addiction treatment. *Addiction*, *93*, 1489–1499.
[549] Marsh, J. C., D'Aunno, T. A. & Smith, B. D. (2000). Increasing access and providing social services to improve drug abuse treatment for women with children. *Addiction*, *95*, 1237–1247.
[550] Minkoff, K. (1991). Program components of a comprehensive integrated care system for serious mentally ill patients with substance disorders. *New Directions in Mental Health Services*, (50), 13–27.
[551] Osher, F. C. & Kofoed, L. L. (1989). Treatment of patients with psychiatric and psychoactive substance abuse disorders. *Hospital and Community Psychiatry*, *40*, 1025–1030.
[552] Swindle, R. W., Phibbs, C. S., Paradise, M. J., Recine, B. P. & Moos, R. H. (1995). Inpatient treatment for substance abuse patients with psychiatric disorders: A national study of determinants of readmission. *Journal of Substance Abuse*, *7*(1), 79–97.
[553] Moggi, F., Hirsbrunner, H. P., Brodbeck, J. et al. (1999)
[554] Weisner, C., Mertens, J., Parthasarathy, S. et al. (2001).
[555] Golden, O. (1992). *Poor children and welfare reform.* Westport, CT: Auburn House.
[556] Swick, K. J. (1992). *A descriptive assessment of project FOCUS' home visit program.* (ERIC Document Reproduction Service No. ED 346962).
[557] Boyd, B. (1992). Impacts of interagency collaboration on participating organizations. Paper presented at the annual meeting of the American Educational Research Association, San Francisco, CA: (ERIC Document Reproduction Service No. ED 346566).
[558] Kagan, S. L. (1991). *United we stand: Collaboration for childcare an early education services.* New York: Teachers College Press.
[559] Raack, L., Kunesh, L. G. & Shulman, I. (1992). *Interagency collaboration in the heartland: Challenges and opportunities. Proceedings of the NCREL Early Childhood Connection Regional Forum (1st, Elmhurst, Illinois, October 14-15, 1991).* ERIC Document Reproduction Service No. ED 344670.
[560] Washburn, N. J., Simmons, S., Sommer, V., Adkins, B., Gerken, P. & Rogers, M. et al. (2006). Outcome of interventions to identify family history and risk management for women with breast cancer in the ambulatory setting. *Journal of Clinical Oncology*, *24*(18S), 6121.
[561] Weingarten, S. R., Henning, J. M., Badamgarav, E., Knight, K., Hasselblad, V., Gano, A., Jr. et al. (2002). Interventions used in disease management programmes for patients with chronic illness—which ones work? Meta-analysis of published reports. *British Medical Journal*, *325*, 925.
[562] Davis, D. A., Thomson, M. A., Oxman, A. D. & Haynes, R. B. (1992). Evidence for the effectiveness of CME. A review of 50 randomized controlled trials. *JAMA*, *268*, 1111–1117.
[563] Weingarten, S. R., Henning, J. M., Badamgarav, E. et al. (2002).

[564] Bukstein, D. A., Jones, C. A., Ledford, D. K., Smith, P., Wechsler, M. E. & Urbano, F. L. (2005). Discussing the COSTS of Asthma: Controlling Outcomes, Symptoms, and Treatment Strategies. *American Journal of Managed Care*, *11*(11S), S318–S336.

[565] Dennis, M., Scott, C. K. & Funk, R. (2003).

[566] Dubar-Jacob, J., Burke, L. E. & Puczynski, S. (1995). Clinical assessment and management of adherence to medical regimens. In P. M. Nicassio & T. W. Smith (Eds.), *Managing chronic illness: A biosychosocial perspective* (pp. 313–349). Washington, DC: American Psychological Association.

[567] Nicassio, P. M., Schoenfeld-Smith, K., Radojevic, V. & Schuman, C. (1995). Pain coping mechanisms in fibromyalgia: Relationship to pain and functional outcomes. *Journal of Rheumatology*, *22*, 1552–1558.

[568] Roter, D. L., Hall, J. A., Merisca, R., Nordstrom, B., Cretin, D. & Svarstad, B. (1998). Effectiveness of interventions to improve patient compliance: A meta-analysis. *Medical Care*, *36*, 1138–1161.

[569] McLellan, A. T., Lewis, D. C., O'Brien, C. P. et al. (2000).

[570] Dennis, M., Scott, C. K. & Funk, R. (2003).

[571] Institute of Medicine. (2006).

[572] McKay, J. R., Alterman, A. I., Rutherford, M. J., Cacciola, J. S. & McLellan, A. T. (1999). The relationship of alcohol use to cocaine relapse in cocaine dependent patients in an aftercare study. *Journal of Studies on Alcohol*, *60*, 176–180.

[573] McKay, J. R., Lynch, K. G., Shepard, D. S., Ratichek, S., Morrison, R., Koppenhaver, J. et al. (2004). The effectiveness of telephone-based continuing care in the clinical management of alcohol and cocaine use disorders: 12-month outcomes. *Journal of Consulting and Clinical Psychology*, *72*, 967–979.

[574] McLellan, A. T. (2002). Have we evaluated addiction treatment correctly? Implications from a chronic care perspective. *Addiction*, *97*, 249–252.

[575] Hser, Y. I., Joshi, V., Anglin, M. D. & Fletcher, B. (1999). Predicting posttreatment cocaine abstinence for first-time admissions and treatment repeaters. *American Journal of Public Health*, *89*, 666–671.

[576] Simpson, D. D. & Savage, L. J. (1980). Drug abuse treatment readmissions and outcomes: Three-year follow-up of DARP patients. *Archives of General Psychiatry*, *37*, 896–901.

[577] Myrtle, R. C. & Wilber, K. H. (1994). Designing service delivery systems: Lessons from the development of community-based systems of care for the elderly. *Public Administration Review*, *54*(3), 245–252.

[578] Reynolds, K. & Koster,V. (2005). *Innovative ways to finance mental health services in a primary care setting*. Washtenaw, MI: Washtenaw Community Health Association.

[579] Davidson, L., Tondora, J., O'Connell, M. J., Kirk, T. Jr., Rockholz, P. & Evans, A. C. (2007). Creating a recovery-oriented system of behavioral health care: moving from concept to reality. *Psychiatric Rehabilitation Journal*, *31*(1), 23–31.

[580] Ibid.

[581] O'Connell, M., Tondora, J., Croog, G., Evans, A. & Davidson, L. (2005).

[582] Ibid.

[583] Davidson, L., Tondora, J., O'Connell, M. J. et al. (2007).

[584] White, W. L. (2007). A recovery revolution in Philadelphia. *Counselor*, *8*(5), 34–38.

[585] White, W. L. (2007). 36.

[586] Ibid.
[587] Ibid.
[588] Ibid.
[589] Barreira, P., Espey, B., Fishbein, R., Moran, D. & Flannery, R. B. (2000). Linking substance abuse and serious mental illness service delivery systems: Initiating a statewide collaborative. *Journal of Behavioral Health Services & Research*, *27*(1), 107-113.
[590] Barreira, P., Espey, B., Fishbein, R. et al. (2000).
[591] Jacobson, N. & Curtis, L. (2000).
[592] Solomon, P. & Stanhope, V. (2004).
[593] Ibid. 318.
[594] Ibid. 319.

In: Recovery-Oriented Systems of Care for Individuals … ISBN: 978-1-62808-648-5
Editor: Jonah Edelman

Chapter 2

ACCESS TO RECOVERY (ATR) APPROACHES TO RECOVERY-ORIENTED SYSTEMS OF CARE: THREE CASE STUDIES*

Peter Gaumond and Melanie Whitter

PURPOSE STATEMENT

This white paper has been prepared as a resource for States, communities, and organizations planning for, embarking on, or well into systems-change efforts intended to develop, sustain, or enhance components of recovery-oriented systems of care. While States, communities, and organizations each face unique challenges and opportunities, the lessons learned by those that have already begun this process can serve as an invaluable resource to other States and communities, offering not a template for action but a menu of options and strategies for readers' consideration. This paper is intended to offer snapshots of promising approaches and is designed to serve as a starting point for discussion.

Using the principles and elements as a point of reference, this document will provide a brief overview of CSAT's Access to Recovery (ATR) program and will describe the activities and operations of three States that have taken steps toward the development of recovery-oriented systems of care through ATR grants: Connecticut, Washington, and Wisconsin.

Despite their varying historical, political, and service system contexts, the projects highlighted in this paper provide useful examples of strategies that might be applicable to other States and communities. Each reflects an ongoing systems improvement philosophy that is an essential component of the endeavor to create recovery-oriented systems of care. None provides a complete template or roadmap, since each State and community is unique, and since in the development of recovery-oriented systems of care one seeks not a static end point, but rather a process of continuous systems and services improvement.

These brief case studies are intended to highlight the unique features of each of the three ATR projects, identifying innovative strategies, approaches, and practices that might be

* This is an edited, reformatted and augmented version of the Substance Abuse and Mental Health Services Administration, Center for Substance Abuse Treatment, dated August, 2009.

helpful to other States and communities as they plan for or implement recovery-oriented approaches.

Overview of Access to Recovery

Initially proposed in President George W. Bush's 2003 State of the Union Address, the Access to Recovery (ATR) initiative seeks to expand the range of addictions treatment and recovery support services available to individuals with substance use disorders through competitive grants to States. In 2004, 14 States and one tribal organization were awarded 3-year grants of up to $7.6 million per year: California, California Rural Indian Health Board, Connecticut, Florida, Idaho, Illinois, Louisiana, Missouri, New Jersey, New Mexico, Tennessee, Texas, Washington, Wisconsin, and Wyoming (SAMHSA, 2004).

In September 2007, CSAT awarded $96 million in new ATR grants to 18 States, five tribal organizations, and the District of Columbia. Awards averaged $4 million annually. Eleven of the 2004 grantees, including the three States discussed in this paper, also received funding in the 2007 round. The thirteen first-time ATR grantees were Alaska Southcentral Foundation; Arizona; Colorado; the District of Columbia; Hawaii; Indiana; Inter-Tribal Organization of Michigan; Iowa; Montana-Wyoming Tribal Leaders Council; Ohio; Oklahoma; the Oklahoma Cherokee Nation; and Rhode Island (SAMHSA, 2007).

As of June 30, 2007, a total of 190,144 individuals had been served under ATR. CSAT has reported the following inception-to-date aggregate discharge data:

- 73.1 percent of individuals reporting substance use at intake reported no use at discharge;
- 23.4 percent of those who reported not having stable housing at intake reported being stably housed at discharge;
- 30.8 percent of individuals who were unemployed at intake reported being employed at discharge;
- 62.4 of those determined not to be socially connected at intake were designated as socially connected at discharge (attended self-help groups or had someone to whom to turn in times of trouble); and
- 85.9 percent of individuals involved with the criminal justice system at intake reported no involvement at discharge.

CSAT has also reported that 48 percent of ATR voucher funding nationally was used to purchase recovery support services. Additionally, 31 percent of treatment providers and 23 percent of recovery support providers for which at least one voucher was redeemed were identified as faith-based organizations (Kopstein, personal communication, October 17, 2007).

Goals, Requirements, and Features of ATR

ATR has three primary goals: 1) expanding consumer choice, 2) tracking and improving outcomes, and 3) increasing capacity. A major focus of ATR is individual choice. The grant requires that individuals are provided "genuine, free, and independent choice among eligible clinical treatment and recovery support providers, among them at least one provider to which the client has no religious objection." They must also adopt vouchers as a payment mechanism under ATR. Vouchers are intended to support client choice by making available a broad array of services. The voucher systems that grantees are required to establish under ATR serve as an indirect funding mechanism, permitting individuals to select from an array of treatment and recovery support services. Direct funding of services by contracts or grant awards between the State and providers is not permitted under the program.

Tracking and improving outcomes and ensuring accountability are also central themes in ATR. CSAT states that "success will be measured by outcomes, principally abstinence from drugs and alcohol, and includes attainment of employment or enrollment in school, no involvement with the criminal justice system, stable housing, social support, access to care, and retention in services." In support of this goal, CSAT requires grantees to "maintain accountability by creating an incentive system for positive outcomes and taking active steps to prevent waste, fraud and abuse."

ATR is also intended to increase capacity not only by increasing the number of individuals that can be served, but by expanding the array of services available.

Finally, ATR emphasizes the use of faith- and community-based providers, requiring grantees to establish "a process to enable providers previously unable to compete effectively for Federal funds to participate in the Access to Recovery program (including some faith-based and community providers)" (SAMHSA, 2004).

The ATR RFP explains the distinction between direct and indirect funding. "Indirect funding means that individual, private choice, rather than the Government, determines which substance abuse service provider eventually receives the funds. With indirect funding, the individual in need of the service is given a voucher, coupon, certificate, or other means of free agency, such that he or she has the power to select for himself or herself from among eligible substance abuse service providers, whereupon the voucher (or other method of payment) may be 'redeemed' for the service rendered. Under 'direct' funding, the Government or an intermediate organization with the same duties as a governmental entity purchases the needed services directly from the substance abuse service provider" (SAMHSA, 2004).

The use of vouchers to purchase unbundled services that can be combined into packages tailored to the needs of individuals offers a mechanism for the development of recovery-oriented systems of care. Vouchers, as they are employed under ATR, represent an approach to flexible funding. In addition, to the extent that they are used to develop customized service packages and to increase choice, they are mechanisms to support person-centered approaches.

Recovery support services are a critical component of ATR. These are nonclinical services that assist in removing barriers and providing resources to those contemplating, initiating, and maintaining recovery from substance use problems. Recovery support services may be specialized and require licensure or certification (e.g., childcare or legal services) or may be in a domain for which there are no licensure or certification requirements (e.g., peer mentoring or spiritual support). Broadly speaking, they can be divided into two categories, those that are provided by peers and those that are not. A peer is an individual who is acting openly as a person in recovery, is explicitly sharing his or her experience as a person in recovery with the individual he or she is serving, and establishes a relationship with the individual served that is based to a significant degree on the peer's experience in recovery.

Under ATR, recovery support services generally, and peer-based services especially, gain a greater centrality than is typically the case in addictions treatment systems. They are not necessarily ancillary since they can serve as the primary component of an intervention that may or may not include treatment. ATR recovery support services include a broad array of services, such as:

- Housing;
- Transportation;
- Food/clothing/basic needs;
- Parenting training;
- Childcare;
- Life skills training;
- Employment coaching;
- Legal services;
- Recreation;
- Service brokerage;
- Recovery coaching;
- Peer mentoring;
- Recovery checkups;
- Outreach; and
- Spiritual support.

Among key challenges ATR grantees face are determining what types of recovery support services to fund; establishing a service typology; selecting and enrolling providers; and developing and implementing performance measures and incentives, reporting requirements, and monitoring protocols. Moreover, the State or tribal authority may need to do extensive training of recovery support providers since many are small community- or faith-based organizations that have little or no experience working with public funders.

Another challenge ATR presents to grantees is the development of voucher systems that operate in tandem with existing funding mechanisms, such as the Substance Abuse Prevention and Treatment Block Grant, State and local funds, Medicaid, public managed care programs, and other sources. Vouchers offer the grantees much flexibility, but they also present challenges related to ensuring integrity and accountability across payment systems and managing administrative costs while setting up secondary payment and service tracking systems.

Information systems are an essential component of the ATR initiative. They provide the infrastructure that supports the many functions required to administer voucher programs. Under ATR, these functions can include providing automated platforms for assessing individuals; tracking slot/service capacity, admissions, and discharges; issuing and tracking vouchers, collecting service and Government Performance and Results Act (GPRA) data; auditing against other funding systems to avoid double payment for services that would otherwise be reimbursable through standard mechanisms; and tracking treatment and recovery support provider performance.

ATR grants provide an interesting case study in the development of recovery-oriented systems of care since they represent systems-change pilots. Moreover, they reflect many of the key guiding principles and systems of care elements identified through the National Summit on Recovery. Among the guiding principles they exemplify are:

- **There are many pathways to recovery.**
- **Recovery is self-directed and empowering.**
- **Recovery is holistic.**
- **Recovery is supported by peers and allies.**
- **Recovery is (re)joining and (re)building a life in the community.**

ATR reflects a number of the elements of recovery-oriented systems of care identified through the Summit. Below are examples of how the program reflects some key elements:

- **Person-centered:** Emphasizing choice and making it possible to create a menu of unbundled services including spiritual supports.
- **Individualized and comprehensive services across the lifespan:** Making available an array of services that can be flexibly deployed to meet the evolving needs of individuals in recovery.
- **Systems anchored in the community:** Relying on and fostering the development of a broad network of community and faith-based providers and emphasizing peer services.
- **Continuity of care:** Creating funding and care management/recovery support mechanisms to ensure continuity across provider organizations and service systems.
- **Responsiveness to personal belief systems:** Ensuring the availability of a variety of faith-based and secular services.
- **Commitment to peer recovery support services:** Relying on peers as an integral part of the ATR service continuum.
- **Integrated services:** Coordinating and/or integrating efforts across service systems.

Each grantee has developed a unique approach to ATR that is specially suited to the populations it elected to target and the service system from which its ATR project emerged. The remainder of this paper describes the genesis and unique features of the ATR projects implemented by the States of Connecticut, Washington, and Wisconsin. In the discussion of these projects, we provide a project-level overview and identify unique and innovative features that may be of interest to States, local governments, provider associations, recovery organizations, and other treatment and recovery stakeholders who wish to adopt them as part of a strategy to develop recovery-oriented systems of care.

CONNECTICUT ATR

Background

The State of Connecticut was well positioned to implement an ATR program. Beginning in 1999, the State Department of Mental Health and Addiction Services (DMHAS), in partnership with the Connecticut Community for Addiction Recovery (CCAR) and Advocacy Unlimited, Inc., a statewide advocacy organization serving persons with or in recovery from psychiatric disabilities and their families, developed "recovery core values" to guide restructuring of the State's mental health and addiction treatment service systems. In developing the recovery core values, DMHAS also hosted statewide Recovery Conferences, established a Recovery Institute and Centers of Excellence, and conducted a series of consensus- building retreats for executive directors, medical and clinical leadership, consumers/individuals in recovery, and several other stakeholder groups within the mental health and addiction service communities. The goal of these sessions was to learn about the views of these key stakeholders regarding the concept of recovery and the steps that would need to be taken for recovery to become the overarching principle that guides mental health and addictions treatment in the State (Tondora & Davidson, 2006).

In addition, in 2000, the Connecticut Governor created a Mental Health Policy Council in response to recommendations issued by a Blue Ribbon Mental Health Commission that the Governor had established. The council, co- chaired by the commissioners of DMHAS and the Department of Children and Families (DCF) and involving 14 other commissioners and key officials, worked collaboratively with the Connecticut Alcohol and Drug Policy Council to drive systems transformation across the State's mental health and addictions treatment systems.

In September 2002, DMHAS issued a policy statement entitled *Commissioner's Policy Statement No. 83: Promoting a Recovery- Oriented Service System* (Kirk, 2002). This document "designated the concept of recovery as the overarching goal, guiding principle, and operational framework for the system of care supported by DMHAS" and committed the State to systems transformation. It defined recovery as follows:

> Recovery is a process of restoring or developing a positive and meaningful sense of identity apart from one's condition and then rebuilding one's life despite, or within the limitations imposed by that condition.

The statement described a recovery-oriented system of care as follows:

> A recovery-oriented system of care identifies and builds upon each person's assets, strengths, and areas of health and competence to support the person in achieving a sense of mastery over mental illness and/or addiction while regaining his or her life and a meaningful, constructive sense of membership in the broader community.

This policy statement emphasized that the service system needed to "address the needs of people over time and across different levels of disability."

Connecticut also developed Practice Guidelines for Recovery-Oriented Behavioral Health Care (Tondora & Davidson, 2006). They emphasize the following principles:

- Participation;
- Promoting access and engagement;
- Continuity of care;
- Strengths-based assessment;
- Individualized recovery planning;
- Functioning as a recovery guide;
- Community mapping, development, and inclusion; and
- Identifying and addressing barriers to recovery.

In a separate policy statement on cultural competence, the DMHAS commissioner directed that the DMHAS system "function with cultural competency that responds effectively to the needs and differences of all individuals, based on their race, gender, age, physical or mental status, sexual orientation, and ethnic or cultural heritage" (Kirk, 2003). The parallels with the principles and systems of care elements established through the National Summit on Recovery are numerous and clear.

Approach

The Connecticut ATR program was conceptualized and implemented within the context of these ongoing efforts toward the development of recovery-oriented behavioral health systems. To develop and implement the ATR program, DMHAS partnered with the State's DCF, Department of Correction (DOC), and Department of Social Services (DSS), as well as the Court Support Services Division (CSSD) of the judicial branch. The State also involved faith- and peer-based organizations, advocacy groups, and State universities in the development of its ATR proposal and in the statewide implementation of its program.

Connecticut ATR prioritizes the following populations:

- Adult women served through the State's DCF/DMHAS Project Substance Abuse Family Evaluation (SAFE) or through the DSS Temporary Assistance for Needy Families (TANF) Program;
- Adults with substance use disorders who are under the jurisdiction of Department of Corrections, on parole, or on DOC reentry status;
- Young adults and adults with nondependent substance use problems who might benefit from brief treatment; and
- Adults with substance use disorders identified through the DMHAS Urban Initiatives in Bridgeport and New Haven (Connecticut DMHAS, 2004).

Initially, the Connecticut ATR program was intended only to serve individuals referred by DCF, CSSD, DOC, or DSS. However, in August 2005, eligibility was expanded to include all Connecticut adults with substance use disorders. Over the life of the Connecticut ATR program, CSSD- and DOC-involved individuals have accounted for 48 percent of individuals served.

Under the Connecticut ATR program, vouchers were deemed the payment source of last resort. ATR funding was only used for individuals who did not have access to entitlements, private insurance, or other resources that could cover the cost of needed services.

Connecticut ATR was implemented and managed through a contract with an administrative services organization (ASO), Advanced Behavioral Health (ABH). ABH's major areas of responsibility include:

- Coordinating authorization for ATR services;
- Facilitating provider voucher reimbursement;
- Managing linkages and coordination of services for recipients while promoting positive treatment outcomes; and
- Collecting and uploading GPRA data in accordance with CSAT deadlines.

ABH also serves as the ASO for Connecticut's State-Administered General Assistance (SAGA) Program, which funds services for individuals who are eligible for publicly funded behavioral health treatment services. The ABH database of services was expanded under ATR to include a full array of recovery support services, including peer- and faith-based services. Use of the ABH database permits services and reimbursements to be tracked across payment sources and thereby increases accountability for services paid through ATR.

ATR provided a vehicle for the State of Connecticut to pilot the establishment of service networks coinciding with its five DMHAS regions. The networks included addictions treatment and recovery support providers, many of which were faith-based or peer-led, and were important in establishing an infrastructure to effectively provide recovery-oriented services locally.

Connecticut's provider networks were established by issuing a request for qualifications (RFQ) through which providers in each region designated a lead agency. The five networks were "defined as a formal affiliation, via Memorandum of Agreement, among…treatment and recovery support providers, including faith- and peer-based providers." They were intended "to provide integrated, coordinated, and comprehensive recovery-oriented…treatment and recovery support services…with continuous monitoring of quality, accountability, and cost-effectiveness" (Connecticut DMHAS, 2004).

The regional networks meet regularly for purposes of systems and services planning and coordination. These meetings have permitted the development of effective partnerships among treatment and recovery support providers. The networks provide the infrastructure to support recovery-oriented systems of care and services under ATR. They also further Connecticut's overall work toward the development of recovery-oriented systems of care.

Connecticut approached both its larger statewide systems transformation and its ATR program at the system, program, and practitioner levels. At the system level, policy was driven by recovery principles and values. At the program level, recovery practice guidelines were developed. Finally, at the practitioner level, Connecticut emphasized person-centered and culturally competent approaches that conveyed hope and respect and conformed to the State's principles relative to recovery-oriented services. The Practice Guidelines for Recovery-Oriented Behavioral Health Care standardize many of the principles that are applied to both ATR and non-ATR services.

The RFQ issued in 2004 to establish the State's five service networks required applicant networks to explain how proposed network providers would "embrace recovery-oriented practice principles and guidelines." These principles and guidelines are listed in the box to the right.

Recovery Support Services

Approximately 85 percent of Connecticut's ATR funding was directed toward recovery support services, including:

- Short-term housing;
- Transportation;
- Faith-based services;
- Basic needs (food, clothing, etc.);
- Case management;
- Childcare; and
- Vocational and educational services.

CONNECTICUT'S RECOVERY-ORIENTED PRACTICE PRINCIPLES AND GUIDELINES

- Fostering hope and recovery
- Encouraging active participation of people in recovery at all levels of the system
- Conveying courtesy, dignity, and respect to all persons
- Promoting the rights and responsibilities of each person
- Delivering person-centered, strength-based, and community- focused care
- Providing culturally responsive care
- Offering multiple entry points for easy access
- Providing a menu of effective services and supports
- Optimizing natural supports and community involvement
- Utilizing best and/or evidence- based practices

(Connecticut DMHAS, 2004)

Recovery specialists (or recovery managers) play a key role in Connecticut ATR. They are often the initial point of contact for individuals seeking services and can provide services prior to, during, and after treatment. Recovery specialists partner with the individual to inventory strengths, identify needs, and determine service needs. They remain engaged with the individual over time, serving as a case manager and working closely with the ASO and with treatment and recovery support services providers. Faith-based providers make up nearly half of the 107 recovery support services providers in Connecticut ATR. This substantial participation is in part the product of work that preceded the ATR grant. The State supported the Saint Francis Academy for Clinical Pastoral Training, which trained hundreds of faith leaders from different faith traditions, denominations, and sects from across the State. The academy is staffed by consultants in medicine, behavioral health, and ministry who provide a spiritual dimension to healing (Saint Francis Care, n.d.). Pastoral counseling services were made available across all five networks under ATR. Among the 38 ATR providers that had no previous history with DMHAS, 32 were faith- based organizations.

Peer services are also a central component of Connecticut ATR. The Connecticut Community for Addiction Recovery (CCAR) has established four Recovery Community Centers (RCCs) statewide and is in the process of opening four more. These centers offer a wide range of peer services (CCAR, n.d.), including:

- Telephone recovery support;
- Family/community education;
- Family support groups;
- All-recovery groups;
- Volunteer training;
- Recovery training;
- Peer-operated transportation company;
- Recovery coaching (CCAR believes recovery coaching is best delivered by a volunteer, usually another person in recovery);
- Referral to recovery housing;
- Employment support; and
- Social activities supported by peer volunteers.

CCAR developed sober housing certification standards and created a Web-based "product that displays recovery housing listings." This enables users to search for recovery housing by characteristics (e.g., 12-Step, Christian), location, ATR eligibility, gender, and so forth.

An RCC offers regularly scheduled "recovery- related workshops, trainings, meetings, services and social events." An innovative service offered by CCAR is the telephonic recovery support program, through which volunteers/persons in recovery from addictions make weekly telephone follow-up contacts with individuals discharged from treatment programs to offer support and to encourage sustained abstinence and recovery. This program has reduced the need for readmission to treatment and has resulted in a more timely return to treatment for those who relapse and require readmission.

In aggregate, housing support accounts for 45 percent of ATR-funded services in Connecticut. Other leading services purchased include clinical (14 percent) and faith-based (11 percent) services and case management (10 percent). The table on the following page shows the percentage of ATR service funding allocated to various service categories.

While 12 percent of Connecticut ATR services were classified as faith-based (e.g., spiritual support), fully 43 percent of Connecticut ATR funding went to faith-based organizations offering a wide range of services, many of which were not faith-based. These services included housing, case management, pastoral counseling and spiritual support. Nationally, 31 percent of national ATR service funding went to faith-based providers.

CONNECTICUT ATR VOUCHER UTILIZATION

Service Description	Percent
Housing	45
Clinical	14
Faith-Based Services	11
Case Management	10
Basic Needs	7
Vocational Services	6
Transportation	4
Other	3

(Trocchi, personal communications, December 7, 2007)

Despite extensive peer involvement in Connecticut ATR, peer-based services represent a very modest portion of services purchased. This is because the majority are reported under aftercare recovery support services (RSS) and other categories. Additionally, volunteers provide some peer- based services, including the peer telephonic support program.

In addition to supporting a range of recovery support activities, Connecticut is also adopting evidence-based practices. As part of an initiative of the Office of the Medical Director at DMHAS, the system has made strides in implementing evidence-based practices. These practices include illness management, RRS for people with psychosis, motivational interviewing, opioid agonist therapy, and supported employment. Additionally, DMHAS is implementing Screening and Brief Intervention and Referral to Treatment (SBIRT) in a hospital emergency department and in a Federally qualified health center in New Haven, Connecticut, and the Matrix Model for methamphetamine- and cocaine-dependent individuals.

DMHAS has also been involved with the ongoing development of provider performance measures. Program and performance measures have been developed in four domains: data quality, utilization, access, and outcomes. Web- based reports are accessible at any time to providers who wish to review their data, as well as information on performance measures across all funded agencies. Training for all providers and system managers on how to use the reports and improve data quality has been provided.

Overall, ATR implementation in Connecticut reflects the three-phase systems-change approach adopted statewide for the transformation of behavioral health care (DiLeo, 2006). It is summarized below.

Connecticut Change Management Process

Phase 1: Determine Direction

A. **Develop Concepts and Design Model:** Perform research and propose concepts and models reflecting principles and core values.

B. **Develop Consensus:** Review concepts and models with key stakeholders, including persons in recovery and agency and association directors. Discuss implications of models for systems and services, resource allocation, and agency functioning.
C. **Dissemination:** Disseminate the consensus concepts and models.

Phase 2: Initiate Change

A. **Focus on Quality:** Institute a provider self- assessment process and require funded agencies to develop agency-wide recovery plans for review and approval. Develop performance standards and measures and monitor.
B. **Workforce Development:** Implement intensive, skill-based training across both treatment and recovery support organizations. Practice improvement initiatives play a key role in technology transfer. Recovery organizations assist in training.
C. **Funding:** Introduce new funding and services and realign existing resources.

Phase 3: Increase Depth of Understanding

A. Describe and communicate the beneficial impacts of the changes on other systems (e.g., criminal justice, corrections, and child welfare).
B. Provide advanced training.
C. Continue developing and improving recovery- oriented performance measures (these measures are currently being finalized).
D. Realign fiscal resources through contract language, competitive bidding, and other mechanisms.

Connecticut and the Principles and Elements of Recovery-Oriented Systems of Care

As noted earlier in this paper, ATR projects generally reflect many of the elements of recovery-oriented systems of care developed through the National Summit on Recovery. However, there are areas where the convergence between systems and services developed under Connecticut ATR and the elements that emerged from the Summit is particularly marked. As our review of the project shows, the following elements are notably reflected in Connecticut ATR:

- **Strength-based:** Using strength-based assessments and recovery plans.
- **Culturally responsive:** Requiring the behavioral health system to respond "effectively to the needs and differences of all individuals, based on their race, gender, age, physical or mental status, sexual orientation, and ethnic or cultural heritage" (Kirk, 2003) as delineated in Policy Statement No. 76 and the State's Practice Guidelines for Recovery-Oriented Behavioral Health Care.
- **Responsiveness to personal belief systems:** Making available an extensive pastoral counseling services network in combination with the variety of secular services.
- **Commitment to peer recovery support services:** Reflecting an exceptionally high level of involvement of peers in the provision of recovery support services.

- **Inclusion of the voices and experiences of recovering individuals, and their families:** Involving CCAR and Advocacy Unlimited, Inc., in the planning of recovery-oriented systems of care and services.
- **System-wide education and training:** Providing extensive education and training to implement Connecticut's Practice Guidelines for Recovery- Oriented Behavioral Health Care.
- **Outcomes driven:** Developing performance measures in four domains (data quality, utilization, access, and outcomes) and training and making a reporting function available to providers and systems managers.
- **Research-based:** Adopting evidence- based practices in ATR, including SBIRT, the Matrix Model opioid agonist therapy, and supported employment.

WASHINGTON ATR

Background

The State of Washington directly funded six counties (Clark, King, Pierce, Snohomish, Spokane, and Yakima) to implement ATR. Each county administered its voucher program with relative autonomy. King County, which includes Seattle, subcontracted with an ASO to implement its program. The other five participating counties worked directly with community-based and faith-based organizations to design and implement voucher programs, to define the array of ATR-eligible services that would be made available in each county, and to determine how best to coordinate and track services. The county-level voucher systems and other components of ATR were built and served as extensions of the State's existing Web-based reporting system.

Washington State dedicated approximately 90 percent of voucher funding to recovery support services. This was possible, in part, because the Washington Legislature increased addictions treatment funding by more than $20 million, significantly expanding access to treatment. ATR provided a mechanism for helping to ensure that this additional investment in addictions treatment provided a return for the citizens of Washington in terms of improved outcomes and subsequent reduced utilization of publicly funded services. To be eligible for a voucher under Washington ATR, an individual needed to:

- Be in treatment or have recently completed treatment;
- Be diagnosed with a substance use disorder;
- Be motivated to actively engage in recovery;
- Earn 80 percent or less of the median income for Washington State; and
- Sign a Release of Information for ATR providers (Collins, personal communication, December 26, 2006).

Under Washington ATR, recovery support services are linked to treatment using a wrap-around services approach. While a wide variety of services were available under the State's ATR program, from acupuncture, detoxification, and childcare to transportation, peer mentoring, and opiate substitution, the State reported that approximately 37 percent of ATR funding provided housing support and transitional drug-free housing, and 27 percent went to case management-related services, primarily delivered by recovery support specialists (RSSs). This allocation of resources was not planned; however, it reflects the needs of eligible individuals seeking ATR services and the relative costs of the needed services.

Housing support, which Washington defined as transitional rental assistance, utilized 30 percent of ATR voucher funding under the State's initial ATR grant. "Transitional drug-free housing," which the State defined as supportive drug-free living environments that provide support services, utilized an additional 7 percent of voucher funding during that period.

WASHINGTON ATR VOUCHER UTILIZATION

Service Description	Percent
Housing Support	30
Information and Referral	16
Other Recovery Services	13
Recovery Support Specialist	11
Transportation	7
Transitional Drug-Free Housing	7
Medical Care (Primary)	3
Other	3
Other Medical Services	3
Childcare	2
Pre-Employment Services	2
Initial GPRA Interview	1
Individual Mental Health Services	1
Other Education Services	1

(Collins, personal communication, December 7, 2007)

Washington State reports that the primary care and other medical services to which ATR afforded access had a noticeable beneficial impact. Consequently, a number of participating counties are exploring mechanisms to continue to make these services available after ATR funding is discontinued. Through the vouchers, uninsured and underinsured individuals gained access to primary care and other needed health care services, including dentistry and various kinds of laboratory work which otherwise would have been unavailable to them. The table below documents service expenditures through the end of the initial Washington State ATR grant.

Approach

Washington State adopted a multistage process for eligibility determination, assessment, and service planning. The process typically begins with a client advocate who performs an initial screening to determine whether or not there may be a substance use disorder and shares with likely clients an informational brochure on Washington ATR. A client advocate can be any clinical or recovery support system representative who responds to an initial request for services or engages an individual who may be in need of services. Individuals who are eligible for ATR services and elect to access them are offered a choice of agencies where they can engage with an RSS. The RSS verifies ATR eligibility, and in partnership with the individual seeking services, develops a recovery plan. Once the RSS and individual seeking services have finalized the initial recovery plan, the RSS issues vouchers to procure the desired recovery support services from the ATR-enrolled providers and refers the individual to a treatment provider for an assessment. Vouchers will also cover treatment services when access to appropriate services would not otherwise be available.

Assessments are completed by a certified treatment provider using a computerized Addiction Severity Index (ASI) and other tools that are accessed through the Washington State data system. The certified provider determines a recommended level of care using the American Society of Addiction Medicine Patient Placement Criteria, 2nd Edition, Revised (ASAM PPC 2R; American Society of Addiction Medicine, 2001).

Washington ATR uses motivation or readiness as an eligibility criterion. During the initial interview, the RSS asks the individual if he or she is committed to recovery. If the individual answers in the affirmative, a partnership is established under the RSS to assist the individual in reaching his or her recovery goals. The partnership between the RSS and individual seeking services is intended to last throughout the period that the individual receives services under ATR. One way in which this partnership manifests is through an open discussion of the best way to utilize an initial authorization, typically in the amount of $2,000 or $2,500, to support the individual's recovery goals. Authorizations are valid for 60 days. Additional funding or additional time in services beyond the 60- day initial authorization requires an additional authorization. The 60-day window was established, in part, to accommodate GPRA data collection.

Statewide, there are about 30 RSSs at any given time, each of whom can have a caseload of 100 or more individuals. While there is some variability across counties, the responsibilities of the RSS are to monitor progress, provide advice or counseling, coordinate care, and intervene at times of crisis. In addition, the RSS tracks voucher expenditures and expiration dates and distributes customer satisfaction surveys. The credentials for an RSS vary somewhat across the six counties implementing ATR in Washington State. In some cases, they are credentialed clinicians and in others they are entry-level workers who have not yet achieved certification. Occasionally the RSSs have been employed by agencies that provide treatment services under ATR. When this was the case, referral rates have been monitored closely to ensure that a disproportionate percentage of referrals did not appear to be going to the organization that employs the RSS.

Washington ATR has not purchased peer services extensively. However, it has relied heavily on a network of over 400 Oxford Houses in the State. A substantial portion of vouchers for housing support has gone to cover portions of stays in Oxford Houses.

Project Successes

Washington State reports that ATR has had a number of beneficial effects. It has led to a more person-centered approach to services in which individual choice and preference have heightened importance, there is greater emphasis on culturally specific services, and there is openness to and acceptance of spiritual support and other services that have not historically been funded. In addition, ATR has played a role in moving the State toward a service paradigm designed to support recovery.

> Washington State reports that ATR has led to a more person-centered approach to services in which there is greater emphasis on culturally specific services and acceptance of spiritual support and other services that have not historically been funded. In addition, ATR has played a role in moving the State toward a service paradigm designed to support recovery.

As Washington ATR moves toward project completion, the State and participating counties are planning for the continuation of services. Some of the participating counties are exploring a 0.1 percent increase in the local sales tax to cover the cost of partially sustaining the continuum of services established under ATR.

Washington and the Principles and Elements of Recovery-Oriented Systems of Care

The Washington ATR project generally reflects several of the elements of recovery-oriented systems of care developed through the National Summit on Recovery. However, there are areas where the convergence between Washington ATR and the elements that emerged from the National Summit is particularly marked. They include:

- **Person-centered:** Strongly emphasizing choice and active participation in planning, including allocating the amount of the initial authorization in support of a recovery plan.
- **Individualized and comprehensive services across the lifespan:** Providing an exceptional platform for the collaborative development of individualized and comprehensive service plans.
- **Systems anchored in the community:** Providing access to an extensive network of Oxford Houses and other community-based housing and recovery services firmly anchored in the community.
- **Continuity of care:** Providing extensive care coordination and case management services, especially through the ongoing partnership between the individual served and the RSS.

WISCONSIN ATR

Background

The State of Wisconsin benefited from substantial planning and systems-change efforts that preceded its ATR grant. The State chose to implement its ATR program in Milwaukee County through a contract with the Behavioral Health Division (BHD) of the Milwaukee County Department of Health and Human Services. Named Milwaukee WIser Choice

(Wisconsin Supports Everyone's Recovery Choice), the Wisconsin ATR program reflects a vision, core values, and a systems improvement strategy that had been in place a number of years before the initial ATR concept was first announced in the 2003 State of the Union Address.

The vision and core values reflected in Milwaukee WIser Choice emerged from the Milwaukee Family Services Coordination Initiative (MFSCI) from 1999 to 2000. MFSCI involved the Wisconsin Department of Health and Family Services, the Wisconsin Department of Workforce Development, and the BHD in a year-long collaborative planning and systems transformation initiative intended to reduce barriers for families involved in multiple service systems. MFSCI fostered cross-system coordination, adoption of a wraparound services approach, development of networks of formal and informal supports, and use of family-centered, strength-based, gender-specific, and culturally responsive approaches (Milwaukee County Department of Health and Human Services, BHD, SAIL Unit, 2007c).

Vision and Core Values

Vision

MFSCI developed a vision and core values through a series of focus groups that included individuals in recovery, service systems representatives, State and local government officials, and other stakeholders. The vision and values were intended to serve as guidelines for systems and services planning and the provision of care. The vision and an abbreviated version of the core values follow.

> Vision: To implement a practice change and system transformation in Wisconsin by having a strength- based coordinated system of care, driven by a shared set of core values, that is reflected and measured in the way we interact with and deliver supports and services for families who require substance abuse, mental health, and child welfare services.

Core Values

Family-Centered Approaches

ATR engages a family defined by the individual seeking services. Family-centered teams and systems focus on the well-being of the family as a whole. (Milwaukee County Department of Health and Human Services, n.d.).

Fostering Consumer Involvement

Families are viewed as full and meaningful partners in all aspects of the decision-making process, including the development of service plans.

Building on Natural and Community Supports

Community resources, both formal and informal, are used creatively and flexibly.

Adopting Strength-Based Approaches

ATR builds on the family's unique qualities and strengths and the resources within its environment.

Offering Unconditional Care

The service team adapts to the needs of the family rather than requiring it to adapt to program models.

Collaborating Across Systems

The addictions treatment, mental health, child welfare, and other systems collaborate with individuals and families to create a single system of care.

Utilizing a Team Approach Across Agencies

All family, formal, and informal team members share responsibility, accountability, and authority, and understand and respect each other's strengths, roles, and limitations.

Ensuring Safety

When child protective services are involved, the team maintains a focus on child safety.

Responding to Gender/Age/Culture

Services are responsive to the issues of gender, age, disability, race, ethnicity, and sexual orientation and reflect support, acceptance, and understanding of cultural and lifestyle diversity.

Fostering Self-Sufficiency

Families are supported in achieving self-sufficiency.

Emphasizing Education and Work

ATR is dedicated to education, employment, and related activities supporting resiliency, self- sufficiency, and improved quality of life.

Believing in Growth, Learning, and Recovery

Team members operate from a belief that every family desires change and can take steps toward attaining a productive and self- sufficient life.

Implementing Outcome-Oriented Approaches

Levels of personal responsibility and accountability for all team members, both formal and informal, are discussed, agreed- upon, and maintained. Identified outcomes are understood and shared by all team members. Selected outcomes are standardized and monitored

Through MFSCI, the BHD identified "the empowerment and recovery of all with mental health and substance abuse treatment needs in our community" as its mission. This vision, mission, and goals, and the core values derived from them, led to a multidisciplinary team approach to services that involved family and other allies in the development of service/recovery plans and in the recovery process. The core values provide an overarching philosophy and common language to bridge formal and informal systems. They also establish expectations that support accountability (De Sousa, 2005). The following key elements identified in the BHD vision statement (Milwaukee County Department of Health and Human Services, 2007) are consistent with the principles of recovery and elements of recovery-oriented systems of care developed through the National Summit on Recovery:

- A behavioral health system that recognizes the partnership with clients, providers, and the community and the accountability to its stakeholders for the effective development and efficient use of resources;
- A recovery-oriented behavioral health system that focuses on the rebuilding of full, productive lives for children, adults, and their families, and supports a full spectrum of services, including primary prevention and early intervention;
- A behavioral health system that attracts, retains, and supports employees and other service providers who are competent and provide excellent quality, as well as culturally and linguistically relevant behavioral health treatment and support services;
- A system in which clients and families are equal stakeholders in service system governance, planning, and delivery;
- A system in which every client has access to strengths-based, individualized, and integrated services that promote health and recovery;
- A behavioral health system where cultural, ethnic, and socioeconomic diversity is valued by providers and clients;
- A vision of behavioral health services and supports that are community based and not institution based; and
- A vision of a behavioral health system that measures its success by establishing and producing clear, quantifiable outcomes.

Approach

Milwaukee WIser Choice serves general population adults ages 18–59 who reside in Milwaukee County, incarcerated individuals who are reentering Milwaukee County from prison, and individuals who are "on probation or parole supervision who are facing revocation proceedings and imprisonment, and who can be safely supervised in the community while benefiting from addictions treatment and recovery support services as an alternative to revocation" (Milwaukee County Department of Health and Human Services, n.d.). To receive services, individuals must meet income eligibility criteria, have a substance abuse or dependence diagnosis, and be referred to treatment. Among the target populations, pregnant women and families with children receive priority (Milwaukee County Department of Health and Human Services, n.d.). The State of Wisconsin requires that at least 50 percent of those served under WIser Choice be from the criminal justice system.

The BHD has operated a voucher program for treatment services since 1994. This program did not cover nonclinical services and was targeted primarily to individuals served under the TANF program. However, because of it, the county already had in place the majority of the infrastructure necessary to support the implementation of the ATR voucher program.

ATR did require the county to implement some changes. For example, faith-based organizations had by and large not served as funded providers for the county. As a result, the county had to establish service categories and enrollment standards for such organizations and then had to recruit them. The BHD also had to create service descriptions and set rates for recovery support services that it had not previously funded.

In Milwaukee County, access to publicly funded treatment and recovery support services is controlled by three freestanding central intake units (CIUs). Two are for the general public and one is dedicated to the criminal justice population. Historically, the function of the CIUs was to ensure that individuals needing treatment were referred to the appropriate type of treatment and that treatment referrals were equitably distributed across agencies. The CIUs served as a triage point, utilizing a brief 30-minute screening process designed to provide sufficient information to make an appropriate addictions treatment referral. Under Milwaukee WIser Choice, the CIUs expanded this process to include assessment with the ASI and placement using ASAM PPC-2R (American Society of Addiction Medicine, 2001). This process takes 60 to 90 minutes. The use of the ASI and ASAM PPC-2R enhanced the CIU screening process, moving it from a substance use screen followed by referral to a treatment agency without appointment to a multidimensional screening process designed to identify the needs of the whole person. In addition, this screening process culminated with an intake appointment at the treatment provider chosen by the individual and with linkage to a recovery support coordinator (RSC), who works with the individual and other stakeholders to build a recovery plan.

While this expanded screening and assessment process was driven by ATR, it was not funded with ATR resources. Milwaukee County adopted the enhanced screening and linkage process for all BHD-funded addictions treatment services and utilized county resources to expand staffing to accommodate the extended process. This permitted the enhanced screening process to be adopted without reducing the rate at which individuals were screened, assessed, and linked with services through the CIUs.

Once the assessment is completed, a level of care recommendation is made utilizing ASAM PPC-2R. Individuals are than given directories of provider agencies to review. Often, the clinician who performed the assessment will assist the individual in clarifying the factors he or she deems most important in selecting a provider (e.g., distance from residence, hours, approach, or faith orientation). Not only do individuals choose a treatment provider, they also choose the agency that will provide recovery support coordination services.

An RSC is assigned to every individual served under Milwaukee WIser Choice. The county has five RSC field teams. In all, approximately 70 RSCs provide services under Milwaukee WIser Choice. RSCs are not required to be credentialed addictions professionals. However, they do need to have a master's or bachelor's degree and are sometimes certified addictions counselors. The average length of engagement with WIser Choice is 4 months, although longer engagements based on clinical need are not uncommon.

Within 24 hours of assessment and linkage with treatment, an RSC begins working with the individual to develop a preliminary Single Coordinated Care Plan (SCCP) based on immediate needs. This begins a strengths discovery process in which the individual's future vision is identified. During this time, the RSC also works with the individual in treatment to develop a Recovery Support Team. This team includes family or friends (natural resources), service system and provider representatives (formal resources), and sponsors or spiritual leaders (informal resources) (De Sousa, 2005). Within 30 days of admission, the RSC assembles and convenes a team consisting of representatives of relevant service systems, family members, and representatives of community, social, faith, or other organizations. The composition of the team is determined in large part by the individual receiving services under WIser Choice. It is this team, in partnership with the individual served, that develops the SCCP. In the SCCP, the client identifies needs and sets goals he or she wants to achieve in the next 6–12 months. As part of the strength-based service plan, individuals in the team meeting may offer to support the client in achieving those goals.

The plan is updated as goals change or needs are met. It provides a recovery-oriented, cross- systems service plan jointly developed by a multidisciplinary team in partnership with the individual embarking on or renewing a recovery process (Milwaukee County Department of Health and Human Services, n.d.).

Through the end of the initial Wisconsin ATR grant, 51 percent of Milwaukee WIser Choice voucher expenditures were for recovery support services and 49 percent were for treatment. Forty-two percent of recovery support service expenditures were for recovery support coordination. Utilization by service category is summarized below.

Wisconsin ATR Voucher Funding

Treatment Services	49%
Recovery Support Services	51%
Ancillary Services	9%

(Sigurdson, personal communication, December 21, 2007)

When recovery support coordination services are excluded, housing services (e.g., room and board, transitional housing, and short-term or emergency housing) was the recovery support service category that utilized the most voucher funding. Community employment services also accounted for a significant percentage of Wiser Choice recovery support funding. The table below summarizes utilization of recovery support services other than recovery support coordination.

Allocation of Ancillary Services Funding

Housing & Related Supports	79%
Work-Related Services	14%
Life Skills Development	4%
Domestic Violence Services	1%
Other	2%

(Sigurdson, personal communication, December 21, 2007)

Project Successes

In January 2007, Milwaukee County reported the following preliminary data on the impacts of Milwaukee WIser Choice (Sigurdson, personal communication, December 21, 2007):

- The total number of recovery support service and clinical treatment providers in the Milwaukee substance abuse network increased from 22 to 170.
- The number of faith-based organizations within the provider network increased from 7 to 40.
- The total number of intakes increased by 61 percent, from 4,318 to 6,945.
- The total number of individuals receiving clinical services increased by 177 percent, from 1,759 to 4,875.
- The percentage of treatment episodes designated as successfully completed increased from 21.3 to 50.7.
- The number of individuals successfully completing treatment increased from an average of 23.6 per month to an average of 145.0 per month.
- The percentage of all clients referred for treatment who presented for their first appointment and received clinical services increased from 40 to 82.
- Sixty-eight percent of all clients who presented for the first treatment appointment continued in treatment for at least 30 days.

Milwaukee County also reported improved outcomes in employment, homelessness, family connectedness, and criminal justice system involvement (Fleege, personal communication, March 28, 2007).

Wisconsin and the Principles and Elements of Recovery-Oriented Systems of Care

The Wisconsin ATR project generally reflects many of the elements of recovery-oriented systems of care developed through the National Summit on Recovery. However, there are areas where the convergence between Wisconsin ATR and the elements that emerged from the National Summit is particularly marked. They include:

- **Family and other ally involvement:** Engaging family and other allies in the recovery planning and management processes. (Milwaukee County Department of Health and Human Services, n.d.).
- **Systems anchored in the community:** Relying on natural and informal resources firmly anchored in the community.
- **Partnership-consultant relationship:** Building services on a collaborative process through which family and other allies, clinicians, and other health and human services professionals work with the individual to develop and support a recovery plan.

- **Strength-based:** Using a strength-based service plan and building concurrently on the recovering individual's strengths and those of the team.
- **Culturally responsive:** Assuring that services "are responsive to the issues of gender, age, disability, race, ethnicity, and sexual orientation and reflect support, acceptance, and understanding of cultural and lifestyle diversity".
- **Integrated services:** Relying on multidisciplinary teams and integration or coordination across multiple service systems.

CONCLUSION

Access to Recovery and each of the ATR projects discussed in this paper embody a significant number of the principles of recovery and elements of recovery-oriented systems of care that emerged from the National Summit on Recovery. As noted earlier in this document, ATR emphasizes individual choice and the use of faith-based and other community- based resources. It also recognizes the important role peers can play in recovery, and focuses on outcomes and accountability. In addition, the voucher program that is required under ATR provides a mechanism for flexibly financing services. Thus, ATR as a whole reflects a variety of recovery-oriented principles and elements, including using person-centered approaches, anchoring systems in the community, responding to personal belief systems, and flexible financing.

Each ATR project reviewed in this white paper reflected the unique characteristics of the service systems from which it emerged. Connecticut and Wisconsin built on prior systems-change efforts, enhancing and consolidating gains made prior to ATR. Washington ATR furthered capacity- expansion efforts already undertaken, enhancing and consolidating treatment capacity gains by complementing them with an array of needed recovery support services. Connecticut adopted a statewide model and used ATR funding to move toward the establishment of formal networks that correspond to each of its five service regions. Washington and Wisconsin, both of which have county-based addictions treatment systems, focused on implementation through counties. Washington implemented ATR across six counties; Wisconsin chose a single county to implement ATR. Connecticut expanded an existing contract with an administrative services organization to implement ATR, whereas Washington allowed each of the counties implementing ATR to decide how best to implement services under the grant. Milwaukee County in Wisconsin elected to contract directly with providers.

States and counties are each unique in their regulations, funding mechanisms, and funding mixes and in the relationships between addictions treatment and other key service systems, such as the mental health, child welfare, and criminal justice systems. This gives rise to unique challenges and opportunities. Across States and communities, different strategies are likely to be optimal for developing services and systems that reflect the principles and systems of care elements. The variety of contexts reflected across the three States studied in this document will provide examples of strategies that may be useful to systems and services planners working in a variety of regulatory and funding contexts.

One theme that emerged across all three ATR case studies included in this paper is the critical nature of the relationship between the vision, priorities, and approaches reflected in the ATR project and two other factors: 1) the organizational, regulatory, and funding context in which the project was implemented; and 2) the planning, policy, and systems development activities that the State or local government had already initiated. Each of the projects reviewed in this document reflected the guiding vision or priorities of the State or county in which it was implemented. Each of these ATR projects built upon, complemented, or enhanced existing infrastructure and initiatives. This may have been important to their success.

By starting with the guiding vision or priorities of the States or communities in which they were implemented, and by involving a variety of stakeholders, including recovering individuals and organizations that represent them, faith-based organizations, and all levels of service systems from clinicians and provider organizations to system regulators and funders, these projects were able to develop the momentum necessary to drive significant systems changes.

Each of these case studies provided evidence that systems change is a process that builds gradually on existing capital, requires support from champions, and is inspired by a vision that is unique to each State or community. It also echoes fundamental principles that are broadly shared across States and communities. They reflect confidence in the ability collectively and individually to improve systems to meet the needs of individuals with substance use disorders.

APPENDIX

Several individuals provided invaluable assistance in the development of these case studies and deserve our gratitude for their time and support in this effort. They also deserve to be recognized for implementing systems-change efforts, which are resulting in recovery-oriented services and systems. The following individuals generously contributed to the content of this document:

Sabrina Trocchi, M.P.A., Executive Assistant to the Commissioner, Connecticut Department of Mental Health and Addiction Services;

Vince Collins, M.S.W., Washington State Access to Recovery Project Director; and

Janet Fleege, M.S., M.A., C.A.P.S.W., Program Coordinator—Milwaukee WIser Choice, Milwaukee County Department of Human Services, Behavioral Health Division.

Also instrumental in the development of this white paper was Andrea N. Kopstein, Ph.D., M.P.H., of the Center for Substance Abuse Treatment (CSAT). Dr. Kopstein, who led ATR activities for CSAT, furnished valuable data for the paper, and ensured that the author was directed to the appropriate CSAT project officers, Carol E. Abnathy, M.S.W., L.I.C.S.W., M.P.H., and Dawn Levinson, M.S.W., who in turn put the author in contact with the appropriate contacts in the States of Connecticut, Washington, and Wisconsin.

REFERENCES

American Society of Addiction Medicine (ASAM). (2001). *Patient Placement Criteria, 2nd Edition, Revised*. Chevy Chase, MD: ASAM.

Center for Substance Abuse Treatment. *National Summit on Recovery: Conference Report.* DHHS Publication No. (SMA) 07-4276. Rockville, MD: Substance Abuse and Mental Health Services Administration 2007.

Connecticut Community for Addiction Recovery (CCAR). (n.d.). CCAR recovery centers in Connecticut: Core elements of a recovery community center. Retrieved March 2007 from http://www.ccar-us/recoveryCntrs.htm.

Connecticut Department of Mental Health and Addiction Services (DMHAS). (2004). *Access to Recovery Program Request for Qualifications (RFQ).* Hartford, CT: Connecticut DMHAS.

De Sousa, G. (2005). *Milwaukee WIser Choice: Core values—how does it work?* Presentation at Milwaukee County Department of Human Services, Behavioral Health Division, SAIL Unit, Milwaukee, WI.

DiLeo, P. J. (2006, December 11). *Recovery-oriented care in Connecticut: From vision to operations.* Presentation at the Partners for Recovery Steering Committee, Bethesda, MD.

Kirk, T. A. (2002). *Commissioner's Policy Statement No. 83: Promoting a Recovery-Oriented Service System.* Hartford, CT: Department of Mental Health and Addiction Services. Retrieved March 2007 from http://www.ct.gov/dmhas/cwp/view.asp?a=2907 &q=334672.

Kirk, T. A. (2003). *Commissioner's Policy Statement No. 76: Policy of Cultural Competence.* Hartford, CT: Department of Mental Health and Addiction Services. Retrieved March 2007 from http://www.ct.gov/dmhas/cwp/view.asp?a=2907&q=334668.

Milwaukee County Department of Health and Human Services (DDHS). (n.d.) *Access to Recovery.* Milwaukee, WI: Milwaukee County DHHS. Retrieved 2007 from http://www.county.milwaukee.gov/AccesstoRecovery9887.htm.

Milwaukee County Department of Health and Human Services (DHHS). (2007, January 22). *Briefing Paper: Milwaukee WIser Choice (Wisconsin Supports Everyone's Recovery), Version 4.* Milwaukee, WI: Milwaukee County DHHS).

Milwaukee Department of Health and Human Services (DHHS). (n.d.) *Single Coordinated Care Plan FAQ.* Milwaukee, WI: Milwaukee County DHHS. Retrieved 2007 from http://www.county.milwaukee.gov/router.asp?docid=9880.

Milwaukee County Department of Health and Human Services (DHHS), Behavioral Health Division (BHD), SAIL Unit. (2007), *Milwaukee WIser Choice Provider Network Directory.*

Milwaukee, WI: Milwaukee County DHHS. Retrieved April 2007 from http://www.county.milwaukee.gov/ImageLibrary/Groups/Everyone/SAIL_AODA/Provider_Directory_complete_New.pdf

Saint Francis Care. (n.d.). Clinical pastoral training. Retrieved November 2007 from http://www. stfranciscare.org/body.cfm?id=983.

Substance Abuse and Mental Health Services Administration (SAMHSA). (2004). *Access to Recovery (ATR) Grants (TI 04-009) (Initial Announcement).* Rockville, MD: SAMHSA.

Substance Abuse and Mental Health Services Administration (SAMHSA). (2007). *2007* ATR fact sheet. Retrieved November 2007 from http://atr.samhsa.gov/factsheet07.aspx.

Substance Abuse and Mental Health Services Administration (SAMHSA). (2004). Access to Recovery fact sheet. Retrieved March 2007 from http://atr.samhsa.gov/Factsheet04.aspx.

Tondora, J. & Davidson, L. (2006). *Practice Guidelines for Recovery-Oriented Behavioral Health Care.* Hartford, CT: Connecticut Department of Mental Health and Addiction Services.

In: Recovery-Oriented Systems of Care for Individuals … ISBN: 978-1-62808-648-5
Editor: Jonah Edelman

Chapter 3

APPROACHES TO RECOVERY-ORIENTED SYSTEMS OF CARE AT THE STATE AND LOCAL LEVEL: THREE CASE STUDIES*

Angela Halvorson and Melanie Whitter

PURPOSE STATEMENT

This white paper has been developed as a resource for States, organizations, and communities embarking on systems-change efforts to develop recovery-oriented system. Each State, local government, community, and organization encounters a unique set of opportunities and challenges when it commits to developing recovery-oriented systems of care. Nonetheless, there are many broadly applicable lessons that can be drawn from the experiences of other States and communities.

Developing and implementing recovery-oriented systems of care are rewarding, difficult, and complex processes. This process is relatively new to the addictions treatment and recovery field, and minimal information is available to guide States, communities, and organizations wishing to develop recovery-oriented systems of care. The case studies presented in this document provide examples of recovery-oriented approaches at various stages of development. By providing a range of examples, States and communities can explore approaches best suited to their circumstances. None provides a complete template or roadmap, since each State and community is unique, and since the development of recovery-oriented systems of care is a continuous process of systems and services improvement. Ultimately, each State, organization, and community will develop recovery-oriented systems of care based on individual needs and strengths.

Using the principles and elements as the framework, this white paper will highlight the activities and operations of two statewide systems and one city system that have taken steps toward the development of recovery-oriented systems of care. It will present case studies

* This is an edited, reformatted and augmented version of the Substance Abuse and Mental Health Services Administration, Center for Substance Abuse Treatment, dated August, 2009.

highlighting work under way in Arizona, Michigan, and the City of Philadelphia. The case studies will describe the following:

- Approaches to systems change;
- Systems and program models;
- Funding mechanisms;
- Challenges encountered, including workforce and training needs, regulatory and other systems barriers, and reluctance to change among key stakeholder groups;
- Research used to inform the approach; and
- Motivating factors and other elements critical to the implementation of recovery-oriented systems of care.

The City of Philadelphia: A Model of Systems Transformation

Background

Historically, the City of Philadelphia's substance use disorders and mental health agencies provided traditional, institution-based addictions and mental health treatment that often reflected acute care intervention models. However, within that broader context, a subset of organizations had been piloting and developing recovery-oriented systems of care framework for many years. These organizations recognized that individuals are capable, with some assistance and a network of supports, of managing their lives without alcohol and drugs. They understood that by providing a recovery-oriented systems of care framework individuals would "increase their capacity to participate in valued relationships and roles, and embrace purpose and meaning in their lives" (City of Philadelphia, n.d., p. 2).

Beginning in 2004, the City of Philadelphia embarked on a process to transform the city's behavioral health system to a recovery-oriented model in which coordination of services and continuity of care would be greatly enhanced. The City of Philadelphia stated the values that would drive its development of recovery-oriented mental health and addiction systems in a white paper developed to support the transformation process. Those values are shown in the box below.

Transformation: The Process of Systems Change

Systems transformation within the City of Philadelphia's Department of Behavioral Health and Mental Retardation Services (DBH/MRS) occurred after a change in leadership. The new director, Dr. Arthur Evans, had extensive prior experience transforming the State of Connecticut's behavioral health system to one focusing on a recovery-oriented systems of care framework. He led Philadelphia on a similar transformation process beginning in 2004.

VALUES OF RECOVERY-ORIENTED MENTAL HEALTH AND ADDICTIONS SYSTEMS

The values of recovery-oriented mental health and addiction systems are based on the recognition that each person must either lead or be the central participant in his or her own recovery. All services need to be organized to support the developmental stages of this recovery process. Person-centered services that offer choice, honor each person's potential for growth, focus on a person's strengths, and attend to the overall health and wellness of a person with mental illness and/or addiction play a central role in a recovery-oriented system of care. These values can operate in all services for people in recovery from mental illness and/or addiction, regardless of the service type (i.e., treatment, peer support, family education).

DBH/MRS leadership dedicated the first few months of the transformation process to assessing the city's existing behavioral health system, getting to know providers, and identifying the needs of the system. Initial assessments revealed that the city lacked a collective emphasis on support for long-term recovery that included linkages between treatment providers, indigenous and faith-based organizations, and other community resources to ensure continuity of care through community supports and institutions that sustain long-term recovery.

Cognizant of the difficulty involved in initiating a large-scale change process, particularly under the direction of new leadership, Dr. Evans and his team first moved to develop consensus among key stakeholders regarding the need for systems transformation. This process began with the development of a Recovery Advisory Committee composed of 25 individuals, including people in recovery and their family members, providers, advocates, and city staff. The first task of the committee was to define recovery for what would be the City of Philadelphia's transformed system. In 2006 DBH/MRS, following the recommendation of the Recovery Advisory Committee, adopted the following definition of recovery (City of Philadelphia, n.d., p. 23):

> Recovery is the process of pursuing a fulfilling and contributing life regardless of difficulties one has faced. It involves not only the restoration but also continued enhancement of a positive identity as well as personally meaningful connections and roles in one's community. It is facilitated by relationships and environments that provide hope, empowerment, choices and opportunities that promote people reaching their full potential as individuals and community members

The Recovery Advisory Committee also serves as a steering committee for several workgroups that have been formed as a part of the transformation process. These workgroups were charged with examining specific topics germane to the development of recovery-oriented systems of care. These topics included trauma-informed services, cultural competence, evidence-based practices, and faith-based services. Under the leadership of the Recovery Advisory Committee, the workgroups were charged with ensuring that their work remains connected to the larger system vision and contributes to its realization.

Recognizing that the City's system had many strengths and that recovery-oriented systems of care framework existed in some areas, DBH/MRS set out to systematize the transformation to a recovery-oriented system of care through a shared vision and common direction (City of Philadelphia, n.d., pp.4-5).

Following development of the definition of recovery, advisory committee members went on to identify recovery values and principles within domains the group felt were important. Concurrently, DBH/MRS conducted a formal system-wide survey designed to identify community strengths and intended to serve as a tool in building consensus and buy-in. The survey asked individuals in recovery, their family members, providers, and recovery advocates to identify recovery strengths within the community. This provided an opportunity for individuals and organizations to highlight their own recovery-oriented activities and afforded the city an opportunity to identify potential models for the rest of the system. More than 3,000 individuals responded to the survey. In addition, stakeholder meetings involving more than 450 individuals from all components of the behavioral health system were convened. The meetings provided city officials with a chance to gather direct feedback about the strengths and the needs of the system and to gather information on views regarding the priorities and staging of the system transformation process. Through this process, the Recovery Advisory Committee constructed a set of priorities for transformation.

The city's behavioral health leaders were committed to the creation of a shared vision and to guaranteeing conceptual clarity. Therefore, the city conducted frequent community forums, conferences, and workshops engaging individuals in recovery and their family members, as well as providers and advocates, in dialog about the vision and the transformation. This principle of a shared vision and conceptual clarity would continue throughout the transformation process. As the process gained momentum, the city invited experts in recovery to present on their work. For example, William White, senior research consultant on the Behavioral Health Recovery Management project, made presentations on the concepts of recovery management and on addiction as a chronic illness to DBH staff, recovering individuals, and providers.[1] He also spoke with members of the broader community, including families and community-based organizations not a part of the DBH/MRS service system.

The Recovery Advisory Committee dedicated approximately nine months to the establishment of recovery values and priorities that flowed from them. Once these were established, efforts were focused on the development of the white paper, as well as a blueprint for change. The white paper, *Innovations in Behavioral Health: An Integrated Model of Recovery-Oriented Behavioral Health Care*, discusses the concepts and history of recovery, general principles of recovery, and the shared need for a transformation to recovery-oriented care for both substance use disorders and mental health. The blueprint, which was under development at the time this case study was written, presents the recovery-oriented vision for the system and describes the process through which the vision, shared goals, and systems priorities were developed. It is intended to encourage DBH/MRS staff, providers, and other key stakeholders to begin thinking about how the priorities and goals of the transformed system will affect their services, organizations, and staff. Each entity involved in transformation will be asked what practice changes will be implemented, as well as what policies and administrative issues will be addressed.

Transformation: What Are the Next Steps?

Moving forward, the City of Philadelphia plans to develop implementation plans that will guide the city and its partners in creating a system that embodies the shared vision and conceptual framework and builds on the resources and models identified through the survey and the many public forums and meetings. System-wide education and training is a top priority in the implementation of the transformed system. The city has developed recovery training to be delivered across the system. This is the first formal training that DBH/MRS staff, individuals in recovery and their families, and providers will participate in together. People in recovery and their families will assist with facilitating the training. The 2-day session will lay the conceptual foundation of recovery and a recovery-oriented system of care upon which transformation efforts will be built. Additionally, an advanced training session is currently under development. The advanced training will help individuals acquire the skills and knowledge necessary to operate within a recovery-oriented system of care. A workgroup is in the process of identifying the skill and knowledge sets critical for individuals providing services within a recovery-oriented system of care.

The city has also released requests for concept papers, asking providers to apply for $10,000 mini-grants to enhance and expand existing services to support recovery-oriented systems of care. The mini-grants will not fund new programs but will instead encourage providers to examine their systems and identify where and how they can infuse recovery-oriented principles and transform policies and practice. The city is also encouraging community-based organizations other than treatment providers to apply for the mini-grants, recognizing that there are many pathways to recovery and that some individuals are more comfortable seeking assistance from faith-based or peer-based organizations or other natural supports. Each of the mini-grant applicants must have an implementation team that includes recovering people. The hope is that these mini-grants will help to raise awareness, increase recovery capital in communities, and develop innovative approaches to system transformation.

As a follow-up to the mini-grants, the intent is to host a conference in which treatment and other community-based organizations make presentations on innovative systems transformation solutions. During the follow-up conference, the city intends to rely solely on the experience of stakeholders from its system for presentations on innovative systems-change efforts and lessons learned.

The city and stakeholders are discussing several other change efforts, including:

- Funding collaborations between providers and people in recovery to develop consumer-run businesses;
- Increasing the number of support groups (peer-run, consumer-run, self-help) around the city;
- Developing a cadre of peer specialists who can team with treatment providers to provide peer recovery services;
- Establishing employment and internship collaborations in which providers and local businesses provide employment and career opportunities for individuals completing treatment;

- Initiating collaborative efforts with Philadelphia community colleges to develop a leadership academy for individuals in recovery. Completion of the academy training would qualify recovering individuals to serve as advocates in the DBH/MRS or in a provider organization;
- Co-locating physical and behavioral health services within some of the city-run health clinics, focusing largely on areas with significant ethnic diversity;
- Sponsoring train-the-trainer programs for people in recovery to assist in continued efforts to disseminate the vision of systems transformation in the city;
- Creating family resource and support centers run by families of people in recovery; and
- Building on the strengths of existing programs that have:
  - employed pretreatment support;
  - demonstrated success by enhancing retention and treatment outcomes; or
  - developed strong, long-term recovery maintenance supports.

Many of these ideas are in the early stages of concept development. However, the process through which they are evolving encourages innovative thinking among providers, community-based organizations, and city staff. Through this process, the city is encouraging providers to think creatively in the creation and adoption of model programs to support recovery-oriented approaches. If an attempted approach is not successful, the providers will not be sanctioned for trying something new. Instead, the city encourages providers to try different approaches based on lessons learned.

> The City is not defining or proscribing program design, giving providers the flexibility to use their internal strengths to create programs and initiatives that will support the vision.

Funding System Transformation

Much of the funding for the current system transformation effort in the City of Philadelphia came from a surplus in Medicaid. DBH/MRS has relied on this surplus to fund many of the innovative programs that have been created. Rather than funding startup or new programs (which can be costly), the city has focused on providing small amounts of money to enhance or shift existing programs to reflect the values and principles of the new system.

Challenges

Agreeing on a common definition of recovery was the first challenge in the transformation process. Because people conceptualize the term "recovery" in many different ways, it was both important and challenging to develop a broadly supported definition. Additionally, consensus needed to be developed and reached on the terms and principles of "recovery management" and "recovery-oriented systems of care."

Providers were initially anxious when the city—their primary funding source— proposed significant systems change and articulated new directions. Early in the transformation process, this manifested as resistance on the part of many organizations. The anxiety among treatment providers and other organizations heightened when the city discussed an all-inclusive process that would evolve over the long term but provided no clear timeframe. Such an open-ended process left many providers uncertain and nervous about their place in the system. All of these challenges were overcome, however, by open communication, articulation of the shared vision at every opportunity, and ensuring that the planning, decision-making, and implementation processes remained inclusive.

Lessons Learned

The Philadelphia experience confirms that building trust and including all voices throughout the process is critically important to systems-change efforts. The city consistently demonstrated a willingness to listen and not make unilateral changes, aiding in the development of trust and system-wide buy-in from providers and organizations. Though there are still providers and organizations that have reservations about the changes, the majority of the system stakeholders support the process and are active participants in the transformation effort. Additionally, the city felt it was important to inform stakeholders from the very beginning that the change process will evolve over time. However, ambiguity can increase stress and resistance to systems change. It is critical to the success of these efforts that any issues that could impede the process be addressed as soon as possible in the planning process.

Summary

The City of Philadelphia has instituted an inclusive process of systems transformation that emphasizes building on existing resources to develop recovery-oriented systems of care.

The city's efforts generally reflect several of the elements of recovery-oriented systems of care developed through the National Summit on Recovery. However, there are areas where the convergence between the City of Philadelphia's work and the Summit's elements is particularly marked. They include:

Person-centered by making the individual in recovery the center of the transformation process. Recovering individuals have been central at each phase of planning and implementation, helping to design the city's recovery-oriented system of care. The city is also developing a menu of services that will meet the needs of the individual, whether the person is seeking support from a recovery-support provider, a community organization, a treatment program, or a peer support specialist.

Family and other ally involvement by bringing families and other support networks to the table as a part of the transformation process. Families are an important part of the city's system, and that is reflected in the various roles they continue to play in the system and in the change process.

Individualized and comprehensive services across the lifespan by changing the system to enhance chronic care approaches and rely less on approaches that reflect acute care practices. The city has also focused on developing comprehensive services that are stage-appropriate and can be accessed by individuals at any point in their treatment or recovery.

Systems anchored in the community through the inclusion of community-based organizations. The city also supports community-based organizations in transformation efforts. This enhances the community support systems and makes them a viable and valued part of the system of care.

Continuity of care by identifying those organizations that are providing pretreatment and recovery support services and enhancing their programs through mini-grants in an effort to develop models for pretreatment and recovery maintenance.

Strength-based by redesigning the system to support treatment and recovery efforts that capitalize on an individual's strengths.

Culturally responsive by reaching out to ethnically diverse populations and supporting recovery in settings where they are most comfortable.

Responsiveness to personal belief systems by including faith-based organizations in the transformation process and in the request for proposals (RFP) process for mini-grants.

Commitment to peer recovery support services by including peer recovery support services in the principles of the transformation as well as by devising strategies to expand those services.

Inclusion of the voices and experiences of recovering individuals and their families by including them throughout the transformation process, as well as by training recovering individuals and their families in peer support and family support activities.

Integrated services by creating an integrated behavioral health care system and by exploring strategies for making behavioral health care available in city-run health clinics.

System-wide education and training through the provision of training and education opportunities from the outset of the process. System-wide education and training will continue as a part of the transformation efforts as the city brings together model programs for conferences and workshops, trains recovering individuals to partner with providers to create systems and services that embody the vision and the mission of the transformation, and provides education to recovering individuals and their families.

Ongoing monitoring and outreach by developing a system that is designed to reach out consistently to individuals and their families and to reengage them in the recovery process through training opportunities, education, and community-based support.

ARIZONA: STATEWIDE SYSTEMS CHANGE THROUGH MEDICAID EXPANSION

Background

Since the early 1990s, substance use disorders services in the State of Arizona have been provided as a part of a behavioral health Medicaid carve-out. Service eligibility is contingent upon financial eligibility for Medicaid. Coverage of all behavioral health services under Medicaid allows the State to offer the same level of services regardless of whether someone presents with a substance use disorder or a severe mental illness. In 2000, Arizona redesigned the State's behavioral health system to shift the provision of service from delivery solely in traditional treatment settings to delivery in treatment and other recovery-based community settings. This system redesign included an expansion of person- and family-centered support and rehabilitation services. A number of factors motivated Arizona to undertake this systems-change effort, including:

- A Federal Medicaid waiver that allowed services to be defined and reimbursed in a new way;
- A statewide ballot initiative that significantly increased the number of individuals eligible for Medicaid; and
- A class action lawsuit settlement that required the State to substantially improve behavioral health services for children.

Peer and Family Support Services

With an expanded array of services covered by Medicaid, Arizona was able to offer a full array of person- and family-centered, recovery-oriented services. Both recovering individuals and their family members were hired to work in the behavioral health system in a variety of capacities. Under Arizona's system redesign effort, recovering individuals play a critical role in providing peer support services (PSS).

Arizona began offering PSS in 2000. Initial PSS efforts focused on services to individuals with serious mental illnesses. However, beginning in 2003, Arizona expanded the focus to create PSS positions to support those with substance use disorders. Peer support specialists serve as mentors and recovery coaches and team with alcohol and drug treatment providers to support individuals in their long-term recovery efforts. A statewide training for peer support specialists was piloted in 2003 and expanded in 2005 to train 65 peer support specialists working in 17 agencies. In 2006, the State achieved its goal of doubling the number of peer support staff, and it continues to expand PSS.

Although the State does not require certification for peer support specialists, several training and certification programs exist. A new training program to expand PSS for people with co-occurring disorders provides training for both treatment providers and people interested in becoming peer support specialists. The 2-day training for treatment providers serves as a guide for including peer support specialists on service teams and trains existing staff to work with peer staff on service teams. Other training targets individuals interested in becoming peer support specialists and provides a mechanism for earning college credit.

Family members are also an important part of the Arizona recovery support service redesign. Many family members are hired by community service agencies (CSAs), which may be nontraditional faith-based organizations and/or community-based organizations. The CSAs provide support services (e.g., health promotion groups, living skills, other family supports) under the Medicaid waiver. Other family members (approximately 181 at this time) provide family and PSS in both licensed behavioral health agencies and CSAs statewide.

The CSAs were added to Arizona's funded continuum of care in 2001. They were created as part of the system redesign to expand access to recovery support services. The CSAs are not licensed and do not conduct assessments or provide treatment, but they are certified through an application process overseen by the Arizona Department of Health Services/Division of Behavioral Health Services, the Single State Authority for substance use services. They are described in Arizona's Medicaid Covered Services Guide as a "natural community support" that uses practical and informal approaches to provide support and rehabilitation services. While many of the services can be provided by a clinician, nontraditional providers often bring personal experience in recovery, shared cultural experience, and other assets that clinicians may not be able to offer.

The CSAs receive both block grant and Medicaid funding. There are currently 12 consumer-operated organizations providing peer services, including depression and alcohol screening, employment training, and educational services for behavioral health consumers and family members. Their efforts have reinforced the focus on recovery-oriented efforts, increasing awareness of what it takes for people to be successful in recovery.

Recovery-Oriented Approaches at the Point of Entry

Within the new system, Arizona implemented recovery-oriented approaches at the front door. In many agencies, when someone enters a treatment facility, the first person they see is a peer, not a clinician. This first contact can be instrumental in fostering engagement with the behavioral health system. This approach has proved successful in Arizona's detoxification programs. Many detoxification clients come into the program with no intention of staying longer than the 24 hours it will take to stabilize. However, when the first person they meet is a peer, they find themselves in conversation and interaction with someone who can relate to what they are going through. This often leads to a discussion about what is next for them, and many find themselves talking about treatment and recovery as something they want or need in their life.

> Arizona's person-centered approach to recovery-oriented services begins when an individual initiates contact with the system.

The assessment process also reflects recovery-oriented approaches. A uniform assessment anservice-planning process has been adopted statewide. It concurrently assesses substanceand mental health issues and utilizes a team approach to develop a recovery plan, which reflects the individual's goals and focuses on building a system of support around him or heThe planning team focuses on helping individuals identify strengths and suppotheir lives and also puts in place a plan to ensthat they will be able to attend the next appointment.

This same planning process is in place for adolescents, utilizing a child and family suteam. The team may consist of a variety of socialservice providers, family members, or a guardian, who provide support for the adolescent. The childand family support team also identifies any urgent issues that must be addressed immediately, such as concerns about the child's safety or a need for prescription medication. There are about 14,000 child and family support teams operating in Arizona, serving a little over one-third of the adolescents in the system.

Community Reintegration

Ongoing recovery support also involves assisting individuals in locating housing and employment. The State of Arizona has worked with provider organizations to provide employment opportunities within the behavioral health system for recovering individuals. It has also provided seed money for consumer-run businesses, including a candle-making company and akeeping business. The State is also collaboratingwith the business community to create job development programs to support employmindividuals in recovery.

The State has developed methods to help individuals secure housing as well. If an incannot afford housing, the block grant will pay for supported housing for individuals and their familieswhile they are participating in treatment. When an individual moves from residential treatment to outpatient services, the State covers the cost of aapartment for the duration of treatment.

Planning for Recovery-Oriented Services

Initially, minimal strategic planning informed systems-change efforts in the adult substance udisorders service system. Systems change was driven by changes in Medicaid that expanded the service availability for eligible clients. The change meant that providers had to provide reimbursable services to Medicaid-enrolled individuals. Providers were challenged withdetermining how to make available this expanded array of services. The State assoffering technical assistance, monitoring utilization rates, setting network goals, anassessing network capacity.

At the time this case study was written, Arizona State officials, consumers, providers, and advocates were in the process of developistrategic recovery plan for adolescents. The document is currently in draft form. The systems-change process for the adolescenservice system has been more structured thaeffort to transform the adult system. The process includes the development of a plan with the support of stakeholder workgroups and defined goals.

Implementing Recovery Support Services

Through utilization review, the State learned that providers were not comfortable with PSS and therefore had not implemented them despite available funding. To increase utilization of PSS, the State convened eight providers to design a peer support model. 2003, the State requested technical assistance from SAMHSA to help adapt the successful peer support model used for those with serioumental illnesses to a model that could be used for individuals with alcohol and drug use disorders. The eight providers piloted the adapted model. The State highlighted the work of the eight providers by scheduling trainings and workshops in which they presented their work. The State also provided $650,000 to expand the availability of PSSwhich then became Medicaid-covered services. Finally, the State developed a protocol for PSS designed to help organizations develop and implement thown PSS.

This creative and flexible approach to funding substance use disorders services has allowed the State to serve more thannly 89,000 people, up from only 8,000 in the late 1990s.

Funding Recovery-Oriented Approaches

Arizona has been able to successfully blend its block grant and Medicaid funding to provide a wide range of recovery-oriented services. While Medicaid accountArizona substance use disorders budget, block grant funds cover critical components not covered by Medicaid, including transitional housing for individuals completing treatment. According to State officials, Arizona had the ability through a waiver to expand their Medicaid service coverage since the early 1990s, but did not systematically identify gapand explore how Medicaid funds could fill thesgaps until 2000.

Challenges and Barriers

One of the greatest challenges Arizona encountered was dealing with clinicians' beliefs at they could control the treatment and recovery process. Medicaid-eligible serviclonger be denied for an individual deemed "not ready" for treatment. Clinicians were acto making many decisions regarding treatment forindividuals, including whether or not an individual was ready for treatment. With the change to the Medicaid-covered services array, providers were now required to provide services for anyone eligible to receive them.

Ambivalence and hesitation among providers regarding the provision of peer services was alsoa significant challenge. Under the Arizona model, peer support specialists have access to clinical records and take part in clinical staffing. Some clinicians initially attempted to exclude them from the staff room and also attempted to prevent them from reviewing medical recordSome clinicians also attempted to hold service-planning meetings at a time when the peer support specialist was unavailable. Additionallin rural agencies, a challenge was encountered when a peer support specialist was receiving services at the same agency where they were providing peer support. Previously there wanothing in a clinician's training that addressed overcoming some of the ethical and clinical issues that they were facing in dealing with peers/consumers as full and participatory members of the service delivery staff.

In response to this, the State developed a protocolto help agencies and clinicians overcome these challenges.

Lessons Learned

Other organizations attempting the same level and scope of system redesign must s se undertake the effort with recognition that change is a long-term and evolving process. Arizona's systems-change effort can be daunting for all parties involved and should be recognizeas such. Any major system shift should include input from all key stakeholders from the beginning. It is also important that all parties—the State, providers, advocates, and individuals in recovery—be flexible and at times accommodating as the process will be continuously revised and adjusted. Cultubarriers can also pose a challenge to systems change.

Summary

The Arizona recovery-oriented change procesan example of how a State can develop innovative approaches to address the needs of individuals and can implement those changes through a long-term and evolutionary process involving multiple parties.

The State's efforts generally reflect several of the elements of recovery-oriented systems of care developed through the National Summiton Recovery. However, there are areas where the convergence between the State of Arizona's work and the Summit's elements is particularly marked. They include:

Person-centered by implementing team-based recovery-focused approaches from an individual's initial contact with the system.

Family and other ally involvement by involving families in the recovery process from the point ofassessment through recovery. Familie provide support services and are valued members of
organizational support staff.

Individualized and comprehensive services across the lifespan by making available an individualized, stage-appropriate, and flexiblemenu of options for adults and adolescents. The systems change reflected the knowledge that the system must change to meet the needs of theindividual, as opposed to requiring the indivto change to meet the needs of the system.

Systems anchored in the community through involving CSAs in the recovery support process, as well as involving community members in community reintegration efforts.

Strength-based by developing an assessment thfocuses on the strengths an individual brings to his or her own recovery.

Commitment to peer recovery support services by the creation and funding of CSAs.

Inclusion of the voices and experiences of recovering individuals and their families by giving peer support specialists a prominent role in the system, employing them in agencies where they are the first contact a client may have with the system, and by valuing their input in thesystem redesign.

Integrated services by implementing the use of an integrated behavioral health assessment. The Arizona system also focuses on assisting individuals in gaining access to community supports following treatment, including housing and employment.

System-wide education and training by msuch efforts a cornerstone of the Arizona systems-change effort. The introduction of peer services required extensive training of provider organization leaders and managers, clinicians, and peers.

Adequately and flexibly financed by creatively expanding the range of Medicaid-covered services and the number of individuals eligible for Medicaid and using block grant funding to provide services not covered by Medicaid.

Michigan: An Evolving Process to Implement Recovery-Oriented Approaches

Background

Michigan's substance use disorders system is operated through a regional structure. The State offices for substance use disorders—the Office of Drug Control Policy and the Bureau of Substance Abuse and Addiction Services—contract with 16 regional coordinating agencies (CAs). The CAs in turn contract with providers in their region and manage the regional provider network. All direct services are provided by licensed community-based organizations. In 2006, the State completed a 3-year restructuring process. This process culminated with the issuance of new administrative rules governing substance use disorders treatment services. The rule change was particularly significant because the State had not modified its rules since they were first promulgated in 1981. Prior to the issuance of the revised administrative rule, State substance use disorders policy and regulation had been driven largely by the requirements of the Federal Substance Abuse Prevention and Treatment Block Grant, which was the primary funding source for substance use disorders services in the State.

Implementing Recovery-Oriented Approaches

State officials began the systems-change effort by reviewing the substance use disorders services and infrastructure with the goal of expanding the service array for licensed provider agencies. Prior to the rule change, the State funded outpatient, intensive outpatient, sub-acute residential, detoxification, residential, and methadone services. With the implementation of systems-change efforts, that standard service array was expanded to include case management, co-occurring mental illness, recovery, and PPS, as well as early intervention. (Previously early intervention only existed within the prevention system.)

The initial change process did not include a vision statement or plan for strategic systems change. The State's environment for the past several years had been one of little or no growth or change. However, community stakeholders pressed for systems evolution. Discussions began to move forward with modest goals. A vision and a strategy began to emerge. When State officials convened a workgroup consisting of providers and other stakeholders to discuss improvements to addictions treatment, consensus emerged that the system needed to be strength-based and recovery-focused. From this consensus, the stakeholders developed values and principles to guide the State's vision and authored a plan to create such a system.

Although Michigan did not make a conscious decision to implement recovery management as defined by the Behavioral Health Recovery Management project and the work of William White, the principles and practices of this project informed the implementation process. Many providers and CAs across the State were familiar with White's work and the concepts of recovery management.[2] Through the multiple trainings he had conducted in the State, many of his ideas had caught on at the local level. Through discussions between the State, CAs, and local providers, the elements of recovery management made their way into State-level systems-change efforts.

To realize the vision that had emerged for Michigan's addictions system, barriers to implementing systems change had to be addressed. First and foremost, the administrative rule had to be changed to allow for reimbursement of an expanded array of services, including case management, early intervention, peer support, and other recovery support services. A State workgroup that includes State staff, providers, and consumers is currently establishing standards for these services.

In addition to designing standards for the State's expanded recovery-focused services, State officials have made a concerted effort to include strength-based and recovery-focused approaches and philosophies throughout the State system. Planning guidelines and documents reflect this effort. Examples include proposed requirements that consumers and families be included in treatment and recovery planning and in decision-making processes at all levels. In addition, the State law governing the advisory council requirements for CAs has been updated to require greater consumer and family participation on the advisory councils.

Training is a critical component of Michigan's systems-change efforts. It serves not only to equip clinicians, providers and other stakeholders to implement new practices but also to support them in adopting new philosophies. Training is an important tool to secure widespread support of the change process. The State has funded several training opportunities for providers, including a motivational interviewing workshop with William White. As part of their ongoing training plan, State officials have requested support from the Great Lakes Addiction Technology Transfer Center (GLATTC). GLATTC provides technical assistance and training on systems-change efforts and technology transfer and continues to work with the State, providers, and consumers on skills training to enhance and support systems-change efforts.

Finally, the State and providers are striving to close the gap between prevention and treatment in Michigan. Historically, prevention and treatment services existed in separate and distinct silos. However, several organizations across the State are working to break down those silos and capitalize on preventionists' community capacity–building skills to support community-focused recovery and relapse prevention efforts.

Among the challenges the State of Michigan faced were fostering understanding and acceptance of new approaches and philosophies and managing the process of change through which they were implemented on a program and system level.

Funding Systems-Change Efforts

Despite the efforts to create systems change in Michigan, State funding is not available to support new services. The State is asking providers to examine their business practices and identify creative ways to reallocate or more effectively fund recovery-oriented services. Additionally, the State is developing strategies to address engagement and retention issues. They have discovered that a significant percentage of addictions treatment funding supports services provided to individuals who enter the system, receive limited treatment services, and then are discharged prior to treatment completion or without linkage to recovery support services. Often a significant percentage of these individuals return within weeks or months. Such "revolving door" services cost the State money but typically do not result in positive outcomes.

Michigan recognized that systems could be put into place that would increase engagement and retention rates, reducing the number of clients cycling in and out of the system. To address these issues, the State has been involved in the Network for the Improvement of Addiction Treatment (NIATx) study to determine which combinations of services produce the greatest improvement in treatment services.[3] This involvement resulted in the State's establishing a policy to facilitate access to treatment by making the initial intake process less intensive and overwhelming for individuals seeking treatment. By implementing practices to increase engagement and retention, thereby reducing the revolving door effect, Michigan believes that it will be able to reallocate resources that have historically funded repeat treatment episodes.

Many CAs have applied for grants to fund recovery support services, and one Michigan CA was awarded a Recovery Community Services Program (RCSP) grant. Providers and CAs will continue to apply for grants to fund recovery-oriented approaches in the State. The State is also looking at how existing, nontraditional community services can be used to support recovery-oriented approaches. State officials believe that even if no new funds become available, changes can be made within organizations to support ongoing systems-change efforts.

Barriers and Challenges

Funding has been identified as the greatest barrier to implementing a recovery-oriented approach in Michigan. However, the State and providers have worked collaboratively to reallocate existing funds to support recovery-oriented services. Additionally, barriers created by the State's infrastructure and administrative codes were addressed through a collaborative process.

Lessons Learned

It is important to identify a vision for the system. Once a vision has been established, values and principles need to be articulated and a structure to support them needs to be developed. It is also important to identify and analyze regulatory, funding, and philosophical barriers to implementation of practices that reflect the new values and principles. A plan should be developed to address specific barriers. The plan may require a multipronged approach that includes statutory and rule changes and statewide training efforts. Without such a plan, systems-change efforts may stall. Finally, the change process will require incremental steps over an extended period of time to implement.

Summary

Systems-change efforts in Michigan continue to evolve incrementally as State workgroups create recommendations to address gaps and barriers. Michigan's ongoing work is an example of systems-change efforts in support of a recovery-oriented approach. It demonstrates how a planning and change management process can become a feature of a State system, providing a mechanism for system improvement.

The State's efforts generally reflect several of the elements of recovery-oriented systems of care developed through the National Summit on Recovery. However, there are areas where the convergence between the State of Michigan's work and the Summit's elements is particularly marked. They include:

Person-centered by expanding the array of services to include a broader menu of choices. The service system now includes case management, recovery and PPS, and early intervention.

Continuity of care by closing the gap between early intervention and treatment.

Strength-based by infusing strength-based principles and concepts into all systems-change efforts.

Commitment to peer recovery support services by adding PPS to the array of covered services in the State system. Additionally, the State has developed a workgroup to design peer support standards.

Inclusion of the voices and experiences of recovering individuals and their families through administrative and regulatory changes. Recovering individuals and their families are now included in many of the decision-making and planning processes, including CA advisory councils.

Integrated services by including co-occurring disorders services in the new administrative rule. Providers are now able to provide these services to consumers in the substance use disorders programs.

System-wide education and training by providing training on systems change and technology transfer. Michigan also conducts a yearly statewide training conference that for the past 2 years has been focused on recovery-oriented approaches.

Ongoing monitoring and outreach by increasing retention rates. Michigan will be able to use money previously spent on "revolving door" clients on recovery-oriented approaches.

Conclusion

The three case studies presented here document innovative approaches that a city and two States have taken to implement recovery-oriented approaches. Systems-change efforts were motivated by different factors in the jurisdictions. In 2004, the City of Philadelphia hired a new director of the Department of Behavioral Health and Mental Retardation Services who transferred lessons learned from a similar effort in another jurisdiction. The State of Arizona, in 2000, redesigned the State's behavioral health system based on several factors: a Federal Medicaid waiver that provided an expanded funding stream; a Statewide ballot initiative that increased the number of individuals eligible for Medicaid; and a class action lawsuit settlement requiring the State to improve behavioral health care for children. In 2006, the State of Michigan began its change process by promulgating an administrative rule change, which expanded the service array. Further, a broader vision for systems change was inspired by community stakeholders.

Implementing recovery-oriented systems of care is an evolutionary process, and the city and States discussed in this paper are at different stages in that process. In each case, the city or State faced unique challenges and barriers which it was able to overcome by collaborating with key stakeholders, including consumers and their families, providers, and other community-based organizations. Despite differences, all three studies concluded that collaboration among stakeholders was required for success. In each study the leaders were able to create buy-in for a common vision and a process for change by maintaining open communication and including multiple stakeholders in the planning and implementation process. The city and States found that entrenched attitudes and beliefs by those involved in the systems created barriers to change and had to be addressed immediately.

Leadership, innovative thinking, flexible planning, and analysis of existing system strengths and weaknesses emerged as key elements of each change process. Another theme that emerged was that change can begin with small amounts of funding or by reexamining current business practices. Additionally, in each case, contributors stressed the need to recognize and commit to a long-term and often difficult process. However, once that commitment is made and all parties recognize that the city or State is prepared to follow through with change efforts, momentum increases.

Despite the long-term nature of the process, these jurisdictions stated that their efforts to move people and systems toward a recovery orientation were worthwhile.

APPENDIX

Several individuals provided invaluable assistance in the development of these case studies and deserve our gratitude for their time and support in this effort. They also deserve to be recognized for implementing systems-change efforts that are resulting in recovery-oriented services and systems. The following individuals generously contributed to the content of this document:

Ijeoma Abrahams-Achara, Psy.D., Director of Strategic Planning, Department of Behavioral Health and Mental Retardation Services, City of Philadelphia;

Christina Dye, M.P.H., Division Chief, Clinical and Recovery Services, Division of Behavioral Health Services, Arizona Department of Health Services;

Arthur Evans, Ph.D., Director, Department of Behavioral Health and Mental Retardation Services, City of Philadelphia;

Doris Gellert, M.S.W., Director, Bureau of Substance Abuse and Addiction Services, Michigan Department of Community Health; and

Roland Lamb, M.A., Director of Addiction Services, Department of Behavioral Health and Mental Retardation Services, City of Philadelphia.

REFERENCES

Center for Substance Abuse Treatment. *National Summit on Recovery: Conference Report.* DHHS Publication No. (SMA) 07-4276. Rockville, MD: Substance Abuse and Mental Health Services Administration 2007.

City of Philadelphia Department of Behavioral Health and Mental Retardation Services (DBH/MRS). (n.d.) *Innovations in Behavioral Health: An Integrated Model of Recovery-Oriented Behavioral Health Care.* Retrieved 2007 from http://www.phila.gov/dbhmrs/ http://philadelphia.pa.networkofcare.org/mh/home/philly_docs/Integrated%20Model%20of%20Recovery.pdf.

Substance Abuse and Mental Health Services Administration (SAMHSA). (2004). *Access to Recovery (ATR) Grants (TI 04-009) (Initial Announcement).* Rockville, MD: SAMHSA.

End Notes

[1] The Behavioral Health Recovery Management project is a partnership of Fayette Companies, located in Peoria, Illinois; Chestnut Health Systems, headquartered in Bloomington, Illinois; and the University of Chicago, Center for Psychiatric Rehabilitation, in Chicago, Illinois. The project seeks to apply the principles of disease management to assist individuals with chemical dependency and/or mental illness to engage in a process of recovery from these illnesses.

[2] Recovery management approaches place greater emphasis on supports within the family and the community that can be capitalized on to enhance recovery initiation and maintenance. Recovery management focuses on the life of an individual and not just the disease. Recovery management recognizes that recovery is an incremental process in which an individual moves through a series of five zones of personal experience and that there is an "ebb and flow" through and across each of the five zones. The zones of personal experience are physical, psychological, relational, lifestyle, and spiritual. The recovery management model uses "progress in one zone to prime improvement in other zones." Additionally, recovery management recognizes three stages in the recovery process: 1) engagement and recovery priming (pre-recovery/treatment), 2) recovery initiation and stabilization (recovery activities/treatment), and 3) recovery maintenance (post-treatment recovery support

services). See Boyle et. al. (2000, June 28), *The Behavioral Health Recovery Management Project: Project Summary and Concept*, at http://www.bhrm.org/bhrmpsummary.pdf.

[3] The Network for the Improvement of Addiction Treatment (NIATx) is a partnership between the Robert Wood Johnson Foundation's Paths to Recovery program, the CSAT Strengthening Treatment Access and Retention (STAR) program, the National Institute on Drug Abuse, and a number of independent addictions treatment organizations. NIATx works with addiction treatment providers to make more efficient use of their capacity and shares strategies for improving treatment access and retention.

In: Recovery-Oriented Systems of Care for Individuals … ISBN: 978-1-62808-648-5
Editor: Jonah Edelman

Chapter 4

PROVIDER APPROACHES TO RECOVERY-ORIENTED SYSTEMS OF CARE: FOUR CASE STUDIES*

Angela Halvorson, James E. Skinner and Melanie Whitter

PURPOSE STATEMENT

This white paper has been developed as a resource for States, organizations, and communities embarking on or strengthening systems change efforts to develop recovery-oriented systems of care. Each State, organization, and community will create a unique design and implementation strategy for recovery-oriented systems of care. The lessons learned by several organizations that have already begun this process are captured in this paper and can serve as an invaluable resource throughout the design and implementation phase.

Developing and implementing recovery-oriented systems of care are a rewarding, difficult and complex process. This process is relatively new to the addictions treatment and recovery field and minimal information is available to guide States, communities, and organizations wishing to develop recovery-oriented systems of care. The case studies presented in this document provide examples, of recovery-oriented approaches within several communities/settings for diverse populations. By providing a range of examples, States and communities can explore approaches best suited to their circumstance. None provides a complete template or roadmap, since each State and community is unique, and since the development of recovery-oriented systems of care is a continuous process of systems and services improvement.

Using the principles and elements as the framework, this white paper will highlight the activities and operations of provider organizations that have taken steps toward the development of such systems. This paper will present four case studies describing:

* This is an edited, reformatted and augmented version of the Substance Abuse and Mental Health Services Administration, Center for Substance Abuse Treatment, dated August 2009.

- The approach used;
- Funding mechanisms used or developed that support the recovery-oriented system;
- Workforce and training issues encountered;
- Research used to inform the structure and programmatic requirements;
- Motivating factors contributing to systems change;
- Challenges or barriers to systems-change efforts; and
- Other elements critical to each agency's implementation of a recovery-oriented system of care.

Agencies used as case studies are Fayette Companies (Peoria, Illinois), and the Behavioral Health Recovery Management Project; White Bison, Inc. and the Wellbriety Movement; the Sheridan Correctional Center Drug Treatment Prison and Re-entry Program and TASC Illinois' role in the project; and the Citizens Planning and Housing Association (CPHA) of Baltimore, Maryland, and their efforts to expand supportive housing in Baltimore.

BEHAVIORAL HEALTH RECOVERY MANAGEMENT PROJECT

Background

The Behavioral Health Recovery Management (BHRM) Project was born out of the recognition that treating substance use and mental health disorders, which are often chronic conditions, with an acute care model is an ineffective and costly method. An acute care model treats intense, sudden onset, short-term afflictions with short-term, time-limited intensive care, and results in discharge with minimal to no follow up or ongoing support. However, substance use disorders and mental illness are not sudden onset conditions like a broken leg that can simply be treated and healed. Instead, they manifest as chronic and relapsing illnesses, much like other chronic diseases such as diabetes, coronary heart disease, and arthritis that require ongoing, long-term care and management. "These [chronic] diseases are often characterized by alternating episodes of stabilization and symptom activation that require long-term strategies of disease management."[1] Unlike the treat and release practice for acute illnesses, when treating a chronic illness, a physician will employ disease management strategies in which the patient becomes a partner in managing the disease. In a disease management setting, the physician is responsible for providing relevant evidence-based medical advice and care including self-care management techniques, patient education, and provider training. Disease management utilizes individualized care plans based on clinical guidelines to manage individuals with treatable chronic diseases. The patient/physician partnership allows the individual to engage actively in his or her care and to live a full and participatory life.

> Recovery management uses the same principles of disease management but shifts the focus from the disease to the individual and from symptom management to building a life in recovery. Recovery management approaches also place greater emphasis on family and community supports that can be capitalized on to enhance recovery initiation and maintenance.

Despite a growing acceptance of the disease management model in the treatment of chronic primary health conditions, reliance on "traditional" acute care models continues in the behavioral health arena. To provide for the piloting of disease management approaches in the addictions treatment field, Fayette Companies, based in Peoria, Illinois, secured support for legislation funding the development of such models. The legislation, supporting a three-year pilot project, passed the General Assembly in 1999.

Michael Boyle, President of Fayette Companies, serves as project director; William White of Chestnut Health Systems and David Loveland, Ph.D., of Fayette Companies serve as associate directors; and Patrick Corrigan, Psy.D., director of the University of Chicago, Center for Psychiatric Rehabilitation, also partnered on the project. Initially developed to create a system change within one organization, the concept of recovery management would eventually influence system change efforts at the State level. The knowledge gathered through this pilot program influenced the revision of the State of Illinois Administrative Rule 2060 to include recovery planning. The recovery management concept would also come to influence systems change efforts in organizations and State systems across the country.

Behavioral Health Recovery Management is the stewardship of personal, family, and community resources to achieve the highest level of global health and functioning of individuals and families impacted by severe behavioral health disorders. It is a time-sustained, recovery-focused collaboration between consumers and traditional and non-traditional service providers toward the goal of stabilizing, and then actively managing the ebb and flow of severe behavioral health disorders until full remission and recovery has been achieved, or until they can be effectively self-managed by the individual and his or her family (White et al., 2007).

Behavioral Health Recovery Management Project

The idea of recovery management flowed logically from the disease management concept. Recovery management uses the same principles of disease management but shifts the focus from the disease to the individual and from symptom management to building a life in recovery.

Recovery management approaches also place greater emphasis on supports within the family and community that can be capitalized on to enhance recovery initiation and maintenance. Because it focuses on the life of an individual and not just the disease, recovery management is broader in scope than the treatment approaches that are most prevalent today. It encompasses social and recreational activities, employment, education, housing, and life meaning and purpose. In a recovery management approach, recovery should strive to be an enjoyable and positive experience.

The BHRM model recognizes that recovery is an incremental process in which an individual moves through a series of five zones of personal experience and that there is an "ebb and flow" through and across each of the five zones. The zones of personal experience are physical, psychological, relational, lifestyle, and spiritual. The recovery management model uses "progress in one zone to prime improvement in other zones."[2] Additionally, recovery management recognizes three stages in the recovery process: 1) engagement and recovery priming (pre-recovery/treatment), 2) recovery initiation and stabilization (recovery activities/treatment), and 3) recovery maintenance (post-treatment recovery support services).[3]

Within a BHRM model, treatment becomes one of many ways in which an individual can achieve recovery. When treatment is necessary, particularly in cases where an individual is experiencing highly severe, multiple co-occurring problems, evidence-based treatment practices are used.[4]

According to the BHRM project staff, recovery management differs from traditional treatment by:

1. Lowering the threshold of service entry for individuals and families impacted by behavioral health disorders, such as working with the existing level and sources of motivation for change, even if the individual or family is not ready to engage in services the clinician would otherwise recommend;
2. Redefining the role of the person in recovery from "patient" to full partner in the recovery management process;
3. Redefining the role of the professional from expert who treats behavioral health disorders to consultant and ally who remains engaged with the individual or family over an extended period of time;
4. Viewing treatment as a multi-tiered intervention designed, operated, and evaluated in collaboration with individuals and families in recovery that also addresses stigma and destructive stereotypes that constitute barriers to treatment and community integration;
5. Shifting the service emphasis from crisis stabilization to promoting the identification and achievement of goals consistent with the developmental needs of the individual and the family;
6. Re-engineering assessment to achieve a process that is global rather than categorical, and continual rather than a service intake function;
7. Emphasizing sustained monitoring, self-management, stage-appropriate recovery education and recovery support services, linkage to the natural resources of communities of recovery, and, if necessary, early re-intervention;
8. Assessing recovery as a multi-dimensional process of personal growth, self-management, empowerment, and self-determination that transcends the biomedical dimensions of recovery;
9. Evaluating service events based not on their short-term effects but on their combined effects on the course of the individual and family's recovery career; and
10. Evaluating recovery programs in terms of a dynamic interaction among persons and families in recovery, service providers, and the community over time.[5]

Implementation of Recovery Management at Fayette Companies: A Shift in Philosophy and Practice

For clinicians who had been trained in and practiced acute care treatment models, the shift to a recovery management approach required training and a conscious effort to accept a significant philosophical change. To facilitate adoption of the approach, Fayette project staff initiated a series of "brown bag" lunch discussions designed to elicit dialogue among project staff and clinicians in the addictions and mental health programs. Many of the discussion topics addressed ingrained philosophies stemming from treatment approaches modeled after acute care interventions. Discussions focused on the chronic and relapsing nature of addictions and psychiatric disorders; others addressed the "power-control" scenarios that are often present in an acute care model. Project leaders outlined the project expectations, core attitudes, values, knowledge and skills in written documents, and also made it very clear to staff that the system and philosophies were going to change. Staff could accept the change and remain with the organization or move on to an organization in which they were more comfortable. Most staff accepted the change.

A comprehensive training plan also played a key role in the cultural shift within the organization. Ken Minkoff conducted a one-day training designed to motivate the staff on treating co-occurring disorders. His training was followed by a series of evidence-based trainings on both substance use disorders and mental health. Training on motivational interviewing resulted in the most significant cultural shift within the organization for both substance abuse and mental health practitioners. Motivational interviewing changed the culture of confrontation and blame that had previously existed in the service units, to one of acceptance, respect, and understanding. It became acceptable for individuals to be ambivalent about their treatment and honest about why they were there --for example, whether it was because they were court-mandated to treatment or because a child welfare worker said they needed to go to treatment if they hoped to get their children back.

Staff was also trained in the community reinforcement approach, contingency management, strengths-based approaches, illness management and recovery, and supportive employment by experts in these areas including, Bob Myers, Nancy Petry, Leigh Steiner, Kim Mueser, and Pat Corrigan and Associates. Collectively, these trainings moved the organization and its staff toward evidence-based practices and a stronger orientation to recovery. They also helped to move the organization toward a person-centered approach in which clinical staff relinquished control over decision-making in the treatment and recovery process, recognizing that the individual or family serve as the ultimate experts and decision-makers in the recovery process. Individuals therefore became partners and active collaborators in the pursuit of recovery, rather than passive responders.

Recovery partnerships became a cornerstone of the recovery management model and reflected the strength-based approach advocated by researchers in the mental health field. The message conveyed to individuals is that the clinician is a partner in the process and is there to help the individual achieve his or her life goals beyond any treatment goals that may exist.

The BHRM project made significant changes in what has traditionally been called discharge and treatment planning. Historically, individuals were discharged because they violated rules or because clinicians determined they were not ready for change.

In the context of residential treatment, Fayette eliminated rules that had little to do with recovery. These included prohibitions on using the telephone or having visitors for a period of time at the beginning of treatment. This blackout period was implemented out of fear that an individual would get homesick, or hear the "call of the streets" and leave. Once the blackout period was eliminated and individuals were able to have contact with their support network outside of the facility, they remained in the program, and the number of people leaving against medical advice declined. Today, when individuals for whom residential treatment would otherwise be recommended decline admission or are unable to participate, they are offered services at a lower level of care. This supports the philosophy of client choice that is so important to recovery-oriented approaches.

The BHRM project found a way to eliminate discharge plans, replacing them with personal recovery plans. In the beginning, Fayette project staff requested a rule exception to replace discharge planning with treatment planning and personal recovery plans. The State later changed the administrative rule permitting treatment planning and personal recovery planning, eliminating the need for a rule exception. Fayette staff started with a treatment plan that transitioned to a personal recovery plan as an individual neared completion of structured treatment and began the transition to community support. Recently, the Fayette staff has developed recovery planning guidelines that can be used from the time of initial intake. They believe these plans meet all administrative rule requirements while still supporting a recovery-oriented system of care. They are awaiting confirmation of this from the State.

Integrated Services

A key principle of recovery-oriented approaches is integrated services. Many individuals served in addictions treatment have co-occurring physical health problems and needs. Many of the addictions treatment clients test positive for hepatitis or HIV. Some are diagnosed with AIDS. The BHRM project works closely with a Federally qualified health center (FQHC) in the Peoria area. Individuals in the addictions program are connected with the FQHC or are linked with other primary health care providers. Facilitating connections to primary health care services as a part of the recovery planning process ensures that the whole person is treated, decreasing potential for relapse that can be triggered by challenges associated with physical health. Recovery support services play an important role in ensuring connections to primary health care and other critical services in the community.

Recovery Support

BHRM is piloting providing recovery support services utilizing recovery coaches to assist women leaving the residential addictions treatment program. Four to six weeks prior to treatment completion, women are offered an opportunity to work with a recovery coach who will assist them in developing a personalized recovery plan. Recovery coaches provide ongoing post-discharge support in eight domains:

1. Recovery from substance abuse;
2. Living and financial independence;
3. Employment and education;
4. Relationships and social supports;
5. Medical and physical health;
6. Leisure and recreation;
7. Independence from legal problems and institutions; and
8. Mental wellness, spirituality and meaning in life.

The recovery plan is developed prior to discharge. Recovery coaches are available to women even if they leave treatment against medical advice. Recovery coaches assist women with their transition to the community and provide support related to the recovery plan. They also assist women in locating safe shelter or housing conducive to recovery, attending to primary health care needs, and support them in working toward a variety of goals, including education and employment.

Financing Recovery Management

The BHRM project continues to receive the majority of its funding from the Illinois Department of Human Services (DHS). Once the initial three years of the project were completed, DHS extended the project for two years and then moved the project from the grant mechanism that had sustained it to the standard fee-for-service contract between the State Department of Human Services and Fayette Companies. Recovery coach services are now billed to either the Division of Alcoholism and Substance Abuse or the Division of Mental Health as case management services. (Medicaid in Illinois covers case management for mental health services but not for substance abuse. Thus, when billed to the Division of Mental Health, recovery coach services are Medicaid reimbursable, whereas when billed to the Division of Alcoholism and Substance Abuse, they are reimbursed using State or Federal block grant funding.) Project staff believe that future funding will rely heavily on demonstrating the effectiveness of recovery management through ongoing data collection. Initial data appear very positive, and the anecdotal evidence also supports the effectiveness of BHRM.

Barriers and Challenges

Initial challenges included rule and financing issues that were resolved through State changes. However, separate funding streams at the State and Federal levels, and the absence of funding streams that support recovery-oriented services remain ongoing challenges. Internal challenges included staff ambivalence and organizational inertia, as well as a belief that staff time was too limited to provide ongoing monitoring and support after discharge.

An unexpected external challenge arose in the form of the attitudes among referral sources for the BHRM project. For example, judges wanted to mandate residential treatment for all referred offenders, regardless of assessed need. Other commonly encountered external challenges of organizations attempting to implement this approach may include:

- The lack of capacity to provide a holistic intervention that treats people, not diseases;
- The resistance to providing services in the community, rather than in traditional addictions treatment programs;
- The lack of systems to blend treatment with services outside the traditional realm of addictions treatment (e.g., vocational, housing, and educational services);
- The lack of coordination between systems, particularly the criminal justice system and mental health; and

- The ongoing problem of getting families and allies involved in the treatment and recovery process.

Two other challenges were raised in providing holistic services. They are addressing trauma concurrently with substance use disorders and viewing substance use disorders from a public health perspective. Viewing substance use disorders from a public health perspective would involve taking a total health approach, providing preventative services, early intervention, and treatment for not only the substance use disorders, but for other health conditions.

Lessons Learned

Based on experience gained in implementing recovery management, the BHRM staff believes the following recommendations will support the Movement toward recovery-oriented systems of care:

- Collect data on the cost of the current system and the cost of diverting individuals to less expensive forms of treatment and recovery supports;
- Track people rather than episodes of treatment and see what factors contribute to recovery and recidivism;
- Promote the benefits of integrated substance use treatment (promote addictions treatment the way education is promoted; for example, it takes a village to raise a child, and it takes a community to help an individual recover);
- Modify State and local policies, rules, and practices that are not congruent with the development of recovery-oriented systems of care (including evidence-based programs);
- Modify addictions training programs at local community colleges and universities to include recovery-oriented approaches and to emphasize compatible evidence-based practices, such as motivational interviewing and community reinforcement approach;
- Integrate criminal justice and behavioral health services (e.g., promote jail diversion policies and continuity of care);
- Promote community-based programs and services that can reduce the need for detoxification, hospitalization, and residential treatment;
- Mandate assessment for trauma in all behavioral health programs and modify treatment programs that lead to high dropout rates for individuals with trauma;
- Connect funding to improving treatment processes and outcomes;
- Track and report outcomes that promote recovery over time (employment, education, stable housing); and
- Promote the growth of housing programs rather than residential treatment (help clients access affordable housing, child-care services, vocational and educational services while receiving outpatient treatment).

Summary

The BHRM project is an example of an innovative recovery-oriented systems of care change effort within an organization. This project is based on the implementation of a specific approach called Recovery Management.

The BHRM project generally reflects several of the elements of recovery-oriented systems of care developed through the National Summit on Recovery. However, there are areas where the convergence between the project's work and the Summit's elements is particularly marked. They include:

- **Person-centered** through a focus on individual goals and plans for recovery. In recovery management, individuals are supported in making decisions that best meet their own recovery goals.
- **Family and other ally involvement** through family and other support from the beginning of formalized treatment/recovery planning. Family and ally supports are an important part of recovery planning.
- **Individualized and comprehensive services across the lifespan** through the configuration of systems and services to flexibly respond to the needs of the individual. Traditionally, the individual was expected to adapt to the norms, requirements, and expectations of the program.
- **Systems anchored in the community** through recovery coaches and other community organizations, BHRM provides ongoing support for the individual in recovery.
- **Continuity of care** through the development of a recovery plan and the assignment of a recovery coach who will support continuity of care for women post-discharge.
- **Partnership-consultant relationships** through the development of the recovery plan. The recovery coach serves as a consultant who partners with the individual in treatment and following treatment to clarify goals and strategies related to the recovery plan.
- **Strength-based** because recovery management focuses on the strengths and resources individuals can bring to bear on their own recovery, not on the deficits of the disease.
- **Integrated services** by providing an approach for integrated treatment of co-occurring substance use and mental health services disorders and by integrating behavioral health and primary health care. Recovery planning also reflects integrated services by looking at the needs of the whole person and linking with a variety of community-based services in support of recovery.
- **System-wide education and training** by conducting comprehensive strength-based training for the staff at the outset of the systems change effort.
- **Ongoing monitoring and outreach** through support over time and continuity from initial engagement through treatment completion through the transition and integration within the community.

- **Research based** through the ongoing involvement of some of the field's leading researchers in recovery management and through the adoption of evidence-based practices such as Motivational Interviewing, Community Reinforcement Approach and contingency management. Research is also ongoing and continues to inform the evolution of the system.

The Wellbriety Movement: A Natural Evolution of the Recovery Process

Background

Native American elders point to the years following World War II and the return of Native American soldiers to the reservations as the turning point for the rise of alcoholism in their communities. The elders believe this trend was strengthened in the early 1950s, when policies moved a significant number of Indians from the reservations to major cities to find work.[6] The move often resulted in isolation and loss of cultural connection, contributing to the increase in alcoholism in Native American communities.

In response to this rise in alcoholism rates, as well as a rebirth of Native pride across the United States in the 1960s and 1970s, the Indian sobriety movement gained momentum. The sobriety movement capitalized on the Native American history of resistance to the dangers of alcoholism, dating back to the first recorded Native American in recovery, Handsome Lake, a Seneca religious leader (1735-1815). By the late 1980s, the sobriety movement that had begun in the 60s and 70s had become visible, and the groundwork for the Wellbriety Movement was laid.

The Native American population recognized the importance of health and healing, as well as the need to address sobriety and wellness through a "holistic way of life involving the family and the community as well as the individual."[7] While some Native Americans did follow the traditional 12-step Alcoholics Anonymous (AA) model, many found the 12-step process culturally inappropriate.

However, Don Coyhis, Mohican Nation, the founder of White Bison, Inc., and one of the founders of the Wellbriety Movement, knew from his own AA recovery experience that there was great benefit to be gained from 12-step programs. He became determined to combine his own healing experience in the 12-step process with Native American cultural and spiritual ways to reach his own people more effectively than 12-step programs alone.[8] By the mid-90s, with the Native American recovery movement fully active, Coyhis and his staff at White Bison recognized that many Native Americans who were seeking healing and wellness "wanted to find sobriety and recovery from alcohol and drugs, and then go on to live lives of wellness and wholeness rooted both in their own tribal cultures and in the mainstream world."[9] It was at this point that White Bison helped to initiate the transition from the sobriety movement to the Wellbriety Movement.

What is Wellbriety?

The term Wellbriety means to be both sober and well. For the American Indian and Native Alaskan populations, the term Wellbriety describes a natural evolution of the recovery processand combines Native American cultural values with the traditional 12-step programs of AA.

Wellbriety is a state of well-being in which the nations can be well only if the tribes and groups are well. Tribes and groups recover only when the families are well. Families can be well only when each individual person is physically, mentally, and spiritually fit.

"Wellbriety means to have come through recovery from chemical dependency and to be a recovered person who is going beyond survival to thriving in his or her life and in the life of the community. To be well is to live the healthy parts of the principles, laws, and values of traditional culture. It means to heal from dysfunctional behaviors other than chemical dependency, as well as chemical dependency itself. This includes co-dependency [adult child of alcoholics] behavior, domestic or family violence, gambling, and other shortcomings of character."[11] Wellbriety is a state of well-being in which the nations can be well, only if the tribes and groups are well. Tribes and groups recover only when the families are well. Families can be well only when each individual person is physically, mentally, and spiritually fit.[12]

Wellbriety: A Recovery-Oriented Approach

Relying largely on the cultural teachings of the Native American elders, Wellbriety is based in the Four Laws of Change for Native American community development. The Four Laws involve family and other allies in a person-centered approach to recovery and are a vital part of every Wellbriety event, resource, and program. The Four Laws are strongly anchored in the community, ensuring that the community remains a centerpiece and ongoing support network for individuals and families seeking recovery. They also demand a level of community accountability, recognizing that the community as a whole cannot disassociate itself from one of its own who is not healthy.

The First Law, "change is from within," "means that human beings must change their thinking, values, beliefs and attitudes before the community can gain lasting healing and a positive direction."[13]

The Second Law, "development must be preceded by a vision," "means that community self-determination is most effective when the community participates in a visioning process to guide its own future." The visioning process asks the question, "what would the community look like if it were healthy and working?"[14]

The Third Law, "A great learning must take place," "means that all parts of the cycle of life—baby, youth, adults, and elder—in a community must participate in a simultaneous learning experience for the community to get well."[15]

The Fourth Law, "You must create a healthy forest," "means that the entire community needs to be part of the healing process from alcohol and drug problems so that the community itself may recover and individuals may become well persons."[16]

The Four Laws of Change provide a culturally-specific view of healing and recovery that is expressed in the American Indian Medicine Wheel. For the very spiritual Native American population, the Medicine Wheel represents the wheel of life which is forever evolving and bringing new lessons and truths to those walking the path. The Earthwalk is based on the understanding that at one point or another, everyone must stand many times on every spoke of the great wheel of life. Until one has walked the path of another or stood on his spoke of the wheel, one cannot truly know another's heart. The medicine wheel teaches that all lessons are equal, as are all talents and abilities. It is a pathway to truth, peace, and harmony, and the circle is never ending, life without end. Within the Medicine Wheel are the Four Cardinal Directions. Each of the four directions represents something different, in the east is success and triumph, in the north is defeat and trouble, in the west is death, and in the south is peace and happiness.

In Coyhis' own recovery, he combined the traditional teachings of AA and 12-step programs with the cultural teachings of the Medicine Wheel. Coyhis placed what he identified as the key principles of 12-step programs on the Medicine Wheel—in the East is healing, in the North is the power to forgive the unforgivable, in the West is unity, and in the South is hope. As can be seen in the Medicine Wheel graphic, 3 of the 12-steps of Alcoholics Anonymous are associated with each of the four directions. Steps one through three, which mark the beginning of the recovery journey through 12-step programs are in the East, which coincides with the dawn and early childhood. The recovery process, the journey around the Medicine Wheel, begins in the East with the first three steps. This helped to provide a culturally appropriate, spiritually familiar context for the 12-step process. A principle of the Medicine Wheel is interconnectedness—all aspects of life are connected, related and involved with other aspects. This reflects the teachings of the Native American culture. "Time and again our Elders have said that the 12-step programs of AA are just the same as the principles that our ancestors lived with one change. When placed in a circle then they come into alignment with the circle teachings we know from many of our tribal ways. When we think of them in a circle and use them a little differently then the words will be more familiar to us."[17]

The Medicine Wheel Teachings:

- Harmony
- Balance
- Polarity
- Conflict precedes clarity
- The Seen and the Unseen worlds
- All things are interconnected
- The honor of one is the honor of all (White Bison, 2007)

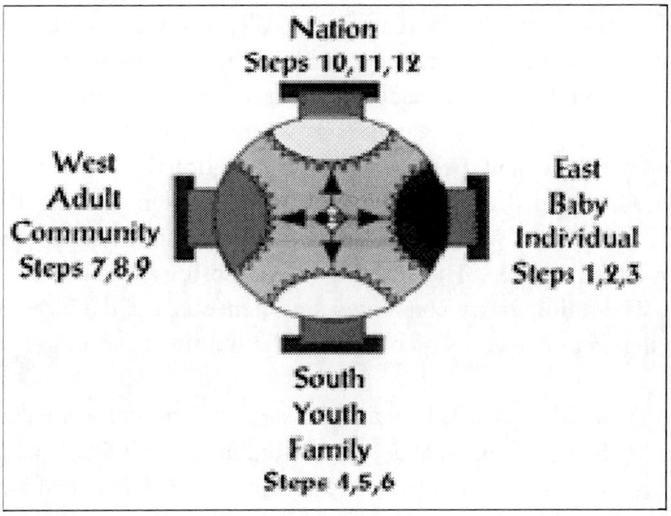

Source: White Bison 2007.

The Medicine Wheel and the 12-step programs.

This idea of using the Medicine Wheel teachings to communicate the 12-step concepts eventually evolved into the Medicine Wheel and 12-step program that was piloted in an Idaho prison with incarcerated males in the early 90s. This approach allowed incarcerated Native Americans males an opportunity to benefit from the effectiveness of 12-step programs expressed in a culturally familiar context. The Medicine Wheel and 12 step programs developed for men gave rise to the Medicine Wheel and 12-step programs for women which were also effectively piloted in an Idaho women's prison.

Between 1999 and 2003, Wellbriety supporters traveled across the United States a total of four times, carrying the teachings of the Medicine Wheel and 12-step programs, and the concept of the Wellbriety Movement to tribes, tribal colleges, and Native American communities. In 1999, the Firestarters program was introduced, becoming a cornerstone for the Native American grassroots recovery movement. Firestarters are trained to work the Medicine Wheel and 12-step programs and commit to continue with the program for four years. Once Firestarters are far enough along in their own recovery, many go on to facilitate their own peer support services, ensuring that the voices and experiences of recovering individuals are included in helping others in their recovery.

The Creator designed the universe Mother Earth to function as a system of circles and cycles. Therefore, to heal we must understand and live by the cycle and circle system in every area of our lives.

spring	summer	fall	winter
baby	youth	adult	elder
individual	family	community	nation
recognize	acknowledge	forgive	change

In order to heal, we must follow the natural order of healing (White Bison, 2007).

Many other programs have evolved from the Wellbriety Movement in response to the needs of different populations within the Native American community. These additional programs are individualized and provide comprehensive services across the lifespan.

The Wellbriety for prisons program has grown to serve incarcerated Native American populations in several State and Federal prisons. Additionally, two programs, a series of trainings and the Coalition Building program, have arisen out of the feedback from individuals who are familiar with the Medicine Wheel and 12-step program and other Wellbriety Movement initiatives. The trainings series brings together in one place several target populations. The trainings are conducted simultaneously and address the needs of every member of a tribe that is impacted by alcoholism. The trainings and target populations are:

- Firestarters (The Medicine Wheel and 12-step programs) for men and women;
- Firestarters (The Medicine Wheel and 12-step programs) for spouses;
- Sons of Tradition and Daughters of Tradition programs (gender-specific substance abuse prevention programs for youth ages 13-17);
- Strengthening our Families (for family healing); and
- Children of Alcoholics (for youth whose families are affected by alcohol abuse).[18]

The Coalition Building, conducted by Community Anti-Drug Coalitions of America (CADCA), teaches Native American tribes how to build coalitions. What the tribe members discovered, however, was that they already understood the idea of coalitions, but for them coalitions were called clans. Tribe members would attend the CADCA trainings during the day, but then in the evening would sit together and transfer the CADCA coalition information to ideas and concepts more readily understood by the clans. The coalition building training program ensures that the system is anchored in the community by teaching, "communities in healing have to band together as coalitions in order to be more effective in accessing healing resources for their communities. It teaches them how to act in unity for the benefit of all."[19]

The most recent addition to the Wellbriety list of program services is called Warrior Down. Warrior Down is a relapse prevention program targeting individuals returning to the community from incarceration or treatment. Warrior Down creates and trains a network of healthy people to support individuals returning home at a critical and often very difficult time in their recovery.

The Movement and its ideas have also begun to spread to other cultures. An African American group is working on their own culturally specific book inspired by the *Red Road to Wellbriety*, the Native American version of the Big Book. The *Red Road* is also being translated into Spanish. The Daughters of Tradition material is being translated into Spanish and Spanish Braille. A sign-language version of the video for the Medicine Wheel and 12-step programs has been recorded. The Medicine Wheel and 12-step programs are also being taught overseas in Australia and other foreign countries.

Barriers

Initially, the barriers were internal and existed within Native American communities that were resistant to change. But now a greater barrier exists in the fact that the Wellbriety

Movement is not grounded in evidence-based science. This has precluded Wellbriety followers from receiving grants from funders that restrict funding to evidence-based practices. Additionally, continued cultural differences plague communications between the Movement's supporters and local, State, and Federal agencies.

Lessons Learned

The most important lesson learned by the founders of the Wellbriety Movement is the need for evaluation from the start of the Movement. White Bison was initially funded by a Center for Substance Abuse Treatment (CSAT) Recovery Community Services Program (RCSP) grant. The organizers chose to spend their grant funds in the communities rather than on evaluation. Now, several years later, the Movement is just beginning to collect the data that can demonstrate, scientifically, that the work they are doing has been effective.

Summary

The Wellbriety Movement is an example of a culturally responsive, culturally literate, recovery-oriented approach. Wellbriety Movement founders saw a need to adapt a culturally inappropriate and ineffective approach to recovery support into something that met the cultural and spiritual needs of the Native American population, demonstrating the flexibility of recovery-oriented approaches to meet the needs of very diverse populations.

The Wellbriety Movement generally reflects several of the elements of recovery-oriented systems of care developed through the National Summit on Recovery. However, there are areas where the convergence between the Movement's work and the Summit's elements is particularly marked. They include:

- **Person-centered** by providing stage and age-appropriate support services for individuals.
- **Family and other ally involvement** by recognizing that recovery requires healing the community including the family, other support networks, and the tribal elders.
- **Individualized and comprehensive services across the lifespan** by addressing the needs of the entire life cycle from birth to elder. The Wellbriety programs have evolved since their inception to meet the needs of all members of the community.
- **Systems anchored in the community** through the Four Laws of Change and the Coalition Building trainings. The Wellbriety Movement anchors recovery in the community and also holds the community accountable for healing itself and its members.
- **Continuity of care** through support for those coming out of treatment, as well as addressing the needs of the family and the community. The Wellbriety Movement offers services appropriate to every stage of the recovery process, including new efforts to spiritually prepare individuals in need of treatment for methamphetamine addictions prior to their participation in a treatment program. Wellbriety does not

provide direct treatment services, though individuals can receive assistance in locating treatment resources.

- **Partnership-consultant relationships** by encouraging individuals and families to seek their own spiritual pathways to recovery and by offering the support services necessary to help them do that.
- **Culturally responsive** through the evolution of the entire Wellbriety Movement. In response to cultural needs, Wellbriety has developed training materials in Spanish, Braille, and sign language.
- **Responsiveness to personal belief systems** through the inclusion of Native American spiritual culture into the 12-step concept to create the Medicine Wheel and 12-step program.
- **Commitment to peer recovery support services** through Firestarter groups that are peer-led.
- **Inclusion of the voices and experiences of recovering individuals and their families** through peer and community supports as well as Firestarter groups.
- **System-wide education and training** through annual Wellbriety conferences that bring together the Movement's supporters from tribes all over the United States. Ongoing training for Firestarters also ensures that those involved in the program are able to continue to provide peer support.
- **Ongoing monitoring and outreach** by making the community accountable. Individuals publicly commit to their recovery in a variety of Native American ceremonies. The community also commits to taking care of one of its own and will return an individual to treatment or to a group if he or she relapses.

THE SHERIDAN CORRECTIONAL CENTER: A DRUG TREATMENT PRISON AND RE-ENTRY PROGRAM

Background

In 2004, the Illinois criminal recidivism rate was 54 percent, the highest in the State's history.[20] To address this historic rate, Illinois Governor Rod Blagojevich proposed to expand the Sheridan Correctional Center to "a national model drug treatment prison and re-entry program."[21] In response to the Governor's proposal, a working group that included community-based providers, representatives from Illinois executive branch agencies, TASC, Inc.,[22] and members of the Governor's staff began to design a system that would address the needs of addicted and incarcerated individuals while they were in prison and provide services in the community upon release. Continuity of care through case management and linkage to community supports for individuals released from Sheridan Correctional Center were intended to sustain and reinforce the treatment and recovery experience. What evolved is a system of care that serves the criminal justice population utilizing recovery-oriented approaches.

> In order to fully support re-entry and the recovery process, services must be designed to holistically address the needs of the entire person including mental health and primary healthcare services, and education and employment goals.

The Design

Identification of individuals appropriate for the Sheridan program takes place at the Illinois Department of Corrections (IDOC) Reception and Classification Center. Participation in the drug prison program is based on security classification, a willingness to volunteer, and an assessment of dependence or abuse. The treatment environment within Sheridan is a modified therapeutic community (TC). However, what sets Sheridan apart from other correctional TC settings is the focus on re-entry that begins on the first day of an individual's incarceration. Sheridan emphasizes a seamless continuum of care that begins with incarceration and continues through release to the community. Clients are connected to services and programs in and outside the Institution that are designed to help them manage and maintain recovery and restore citizenship. The focus on restoring citizenship requires that the services within the Sheridan system go beyond substance use disorder treatment. To fully support re-entry and the recovery process, services must be designed to holistically address the needs of the entire person including mental health and primary healthcare services, and education and employment goals.

The Sheridan program is also committed to peer recovery support services. These are offered in the prison through a peer-led support group known as the Inner Circle. Inner Circle is intended to support incarcerated individuals who wish to enter recovery and to stay crime free following their release. This group meets weekly inside Sheridan and provides opportunities for individuals to share concerns and support and to help each other develop plans for returning to the community. Upon release, Inner Circle participants join a Winners' Circle group, which serves a similar function in the community. This ongoing peer recovery support is a critical component of the Sheridan model.

Winners' Circle is a peer-led, peer-driven support group designed to address the special needs of formerly incarcerated individuals. Membership is open to formerly incarcerated individuals, as well as their families, friends, and allies. Participants must express a desire to participate in their own healing and recovery. They must also be committed to assisting others through encouragement and support. Winners' Circle events provide a positive, social setting in which participants can explore and develop new life skills in a relaxed and non-judgmental setting.[23]

Return to the Community: The Need for Linkages and Community Supports

Because individuals take part in treatment for six to nine months, over half return to the community and are able to "step-down" into a supportive living arrangement. This can include transitional housing, halfway houses, or recovery homes. Many parolees require employment and education support services as a part of their re-entry plan. The continuity of care from incarceration to release allows continued access to services that will help them meet their employment and education goals.

TASC and the parole system work closely together to support an individual's re-entry into the community. TASC provides clinical re-entry case management, intensive case management services specially designed for offenders returning to the community,[24] and the parole system provides supervision and enforcement. Unique to the parole system, TASC and the parole staff devise creative strategies to provide incentives and sanctions in support of the parolee recovery and successful re-entry. Historically, when a releasee relapsed or stopped attending mandated treatment, he or she would be deemed in violation of parole and sent back to the correctional system. This resulted in high recidivism rates and reflected a failure to recognize the chronic and relapsing nature of addictions. With clinical re-entry case management, sanctions do not include an automatic return to prison for an individual. When relapse occurs or potential relapse issues are identified, a group consisting of the parolee, family members, TASC, a member of parole, other community-service providers, and the treatment provider develop a plan to address the relapse and to respond to factors that may have contributed to the relapse episode, such as continued unemployment, lack of adequate housing, or lack of child care. Then together, in a client-centered, community support process, the group identifies strategies to resolve those issues. However, while case management and creative sanctions and incentives play an important role in decreasing recidivism and supporting individuals seeking recovery, the parolee's return to family and community is stressful and may lead to relapse.

Multiple studies suggest that the point of return to family and/or community is a critical juncture of vulnerability to relapse and consequently, re-incarceration. Communities often reject individuals returning from incarceration out of mistrust and fear that the parolee will re-offend.

> A blended funding stream pays for the services provided post-release through the Sheridan Project. Multiple funding sources allow individuals to access a range of services critical to their successful re-entry and recovery.

Key stakeholders in the Sheridan project brainstormed a way to address this juncture of vulnerability in a manner that built support capacity in the community. Their solution was to create Community Support Advisory Councils (CSACs), which are intended to assist recovering parolees in (re)joining the community and (re)building a life in it. CSACs are composed of individuals who live and work in high-impact communities and include community service providers, employers, and faith-based organizations of a variety of denominations. They engage offenders prior to release to ensure continuity of support. CSACs adopt a client-centered approach and strive to serve as the face of re-entry for the recovering parolees returning to the community. CSACs also serve as a buffer between an often unsupportive or hostile community and the parolee.

Financing Re-entry and Recovery Following Incarceration

A critical system element of recovery-oriented systems of care is that they be adequately and flexibly financed. The Sheridan project is funded through IDOC, which has woven together a creative funding strategy that has been essential to the success of the program. A blended funding stream pays for most of the services that an individual receives upon release from incarceration, including mental health care and housing. The multiple funding streams afford parolees access to a variety of services critical to successful re-entry and recovery.

However, the flexible funding comes with its own set of challenges. Each of the blended funding streams entails separate reporting requirements, application processes, and timelines, making record keeping, reporting, and fiscal management challenging, though not insurmountable.

Other Challenges

Collaborations, though highly effective, are difficult to maintain. The collaboration essential to Sheridan's success experienced a number of challenges, many of which had to do with conflicting regulations, procedures, and priorities across systems. However, strong leadership from the Governor's staff helped to overcome many of the cross-system challenges. In addition, giving key staff from each participating State agency a voice in the process helped ensure that there was buy-in to the project across agencies. This created an environment where conflict collaboration, and trust among all parties, resolution was feasible. An example of a including the offender and his or her family. situation in which conflict was engendered by cross-systems collaboration emerged in the Sheridan TC. Typically, within an IDOC Institution, the treatment staff schedule the entire day for inmates participating in the TC. In the Sheridan project, however, a variety of services competed with the traditional TC activities. These included academic and job training classes, clinical interdisciplinary case staffings, and Inner Circle meetings. Negotiating room in the schedule for all of the support services created an unexpected challenge.

Other challenges included securing immediate employment for individuals returning to the community. A related challenge is that an individual recently released from a drug treatment prison may be tempted to use substances again with the money from his first paycheck. Finally, overcoming many of the historical philosophical beliefs and practices within the parole system posed challenges. For example, individuals released from prison cannot move from the address to which they were released until parole makes contact. This could take three days or more. If the individual has a treatment appointment the day of or the day following release, this poses a challenge for the TASC staff member who wants to get that person into community-based treatment immediately. TASC could not move the individual or he would be in violation of his parole.

None of the challenges were insurmountable. Addressing them, however, required strong leadership, and timely communication, collaboration, and trust among all parties, including the offender and his or her family.

Lessons Learned

Designing the right evaluation from the inception of the project is important. This requires articulating goals, benchmarks, and thresholds during the planning process. Strong leadership is essential to the success of the project. Leadership must be able to bring the right individuals and systems to the table to frankly discuss systems change issues before, during, and after implementation. In designing a recovery-oriented system that works with individuals whose relapse could hinge on split second decisions or responses, rapid and real time communication is essential. Trust, openness, and a willingness to take risks are also essential in creating systems change. To be effective, everybody has to share common goals. In a recovery-oriented system of care for offenders, there also must be a focus on community capacity building, restorative justice, and reintegration of returning offenders into families and communities. This requires changes in communities, not just the individual.

Summary

The Sheridan Correctional Center drug treatment prison and re-entry initiative is an example of a systems-change effort intended to develop recovery-oriented systems of care serving offenders returning to the community from prison. Because of the high rates of drug use and related recidivism for the non-violent, incarcerated population, creating a recovery-oriented approach to support incarcerated individuals is an important step towards eliminating the continuing cycle of drug related offenses. Building recovery-oriented systems of care for parolees has the potential to reduce recidivism, saving tax payers money. It also contributes to the health and safety of the community.

The Sheridan Project generally reflects several of the elements of recovery-oriented systems of care developed through the National Summit on Recovery. However, there are areas where the convergence between the Project's work and the Summit's elements is particularly marked. They include:

- **Family and other ally involvement** through support services offered for both the family and the parolee in coordination with the CSACs, TASC and parole.
- **Systems anchored in the community** through the ongoing community advocacy work of the CSACs. The CSACs provide an anchor to community support services for returning individuals and their families. TASC and other support providers also connect individuals to community-based support services including treatment, and education and employment programs.
- **Continuity of care** through case management services that begin prior to release from incarceration as well as through the work of the CSACs that reach into the Institution and connect with individuals prior to their release.
- **Commitment to peer recovery support services** through Inner Circles inside the Institution and Winners' Circles within the community following release. Both of these groups rely on peers to support individuals throughout the incarceration, release, and recovery process.

- **Inclusion of the voices and experiences of recovering individuals and their families** through the use of Winners' Circles and CSACs in supporting individuals in their recovery.
- **Integrated services** through an array of community support services. The needs of individuals returning to the community are broad and include housing, employment, education, transportation, and child care. These services are integrated through the ongoing communication and advocacy of the CSACs and community support providers.
- **Ongoing monitoring and outreach** through continued and coordinated case management services provided by TASC.
- **Adequately and flexibly financed** by creatively blending multiple funding streams to access services that traditionally have not been financed by the Department of Corrections.

Building Support for Supportive Recovery Housing: The Citizens Planning and Housing Association of Baltimore

Background

Facilitating and sustaining recovery efforts in many communities across the country is dependent upon safe and secure housing. Upon completion of substance use treatment, many individuals need supportive housing and have few available housing options. Like many cities, the City of Baltimore lacked safe affordable housing. For those without housing, the primary housing alternative was often living in crowded community shelters or returning to their former living environments that contributed to their addiction, thus starting the cycle of addiction all over again. In 2005, a small group of community organizers working at the Citizens Planning and Housing Association (CPHA) of Baltimore launched a plan to address the housing situation for recovering individuals.

CPHA is a community organizing citizen action organization with a sixty year history of facilitating citizen action around neighborhood stabilization, leadership development, public transportation, and capacity building. They also helped craft some of the first fair housing legislation in the country. CPHA assists grass-roots neighborhood organizations, fostering collaboration and coordinated action to achieve shared goals. Composed of an executive director, a lead organizer, five special interest organizers, two support staff and student interns from the University of Maryland School of Social Work, CPHA spearheaded their supportive housing recovery initiative.

Supportive Housing

These group living arrangements provide residents with housing and support commonly found in a family unit. Residents adhere to house rules and participate in similar activities, e.g., meal preparation, house and property maintenance and gainful employment when possible. The supportive housing model also serves as a bridge for family reunification, encouraging residents to address past problems that have been neglected, e.g., children in foster care, unpaid child support, and damaged family relationships. Utilizing the Twelve-Step model, residents of supportive housing programs begin repairing relationships with family and significant others. Most supportive houses have designated times (usually weekends) for family visits. Supportive housing is not subject to State licensure or certification, because services which require licensure are not provided.[25]

In Baltimore, Maryland, supportive housing was needed to support the recovery process where there was a scarcity of affordable housing and insufficient residential treatment beds in the City's existing addictions continuum of care. Preliminary research estimated 18,000-20,000 treatment admissions annually in Baltimore with only 450 available city residential treatment beds. Historically, there had been widespread community-level opposition to the placement of supportive housing and addictions treatment facilities in neighborhoods. Frequently, such dwellings were denied building permits or forced out of communities where they were already operating.

The Process of Building Support

While the addictions treatment system in Baltimore had begun to recognize the need for more recovery-oriented approaches to care, widespread stigma remained an obstacle to the development of services in the community, including housing. Aware of misperceptions and stigma associated with supportive housing in the City, CPHA decided to address the communication gap and the resistance to placement of supportive housing and treatment programs in local neighborhoods. The lack of communication and collaboration among treatment providers, supportive housing operators, and community stakeholders was having a detrimental affect on the community, and CPHA hoped to bridge the communication disconnect that divided these groups.

Multiple issues needed to be addressed for collaboration to occur. Community residents were concerned about the lack of State and local regulatory oversight of certain kinds, "unlicensed recovery homes" of supportive housing. Reports circulated about overcrowding, inappropriate activities, and public incidents/disturbances involving supportive housing residents.

As was stated, supportive housing is not licensed in Maryland, and staff who work in the homes are not credentialed. This created a belief by many treatment providers that supportive housing did not effectively support recovering individuals. Finally, there was the perceived unwillingness of the supportive housing operators, who embraced an abstinence-based philosophy, to accommodate individuals receiving methadone or participating in other medically-assisted treatment approaches. Many of the supportive housing operators were in recovery themselves and at odds with different pathways to recovery.

Initiating Dialogue

Beginning in July 2004, the CPHA Drug Treatment Committee began a series of "Hot Topics" educational forums targeting treatment and zoning reform. Treatment providers, community stakeholders, supportive housing operators, and key city officials were invited as guest speakers to these forums.

Participants represented the Mayor's Office of Neighborhoods, the City Planning Department, Baltimore Substance Abuse Systems (BSAS), the University of Maryland Drug Policy Clinic, members of The Baltimore City Council and Community Housing Association members. Over 80 participants attended the initial meeting held at the University of Maryland Law School. While the agenda included bills before the City Council regarding licensed group homes and outpatient treatment facilities, unlicensed group "recovery homes" (as they were called at the time) dominated the discussions. The outgrowth of the forums was the creation of a more common vision among the various stakeholder groups regarding the value of group recovery homes and their designation as supportive housing. For purposes of this report, we will refer to supportive homes for residents in recovery as "supportive recovery homes/housing."

In late 2004, Baltimore City Council adopted Bill 04-1555 for the purpose of establishing a Supportive Housing Task Force to study the operations and code enforcement of the homes to ensure safe conditions for supportive housing residents and the neighborhoods that surrounded them. Composed of four subcommittees, legal, funding, best practices, operations and enforcement, the Task Force met regularly from December 2004, through February 2005, and developed an increased understanding related to supportive "recovery" homes.

Another important outcome was a proposal with three core recommendations:

- Development and dissemination of educational materials pertaining to supportive housing;
- Development of a one-stop system for "problem" properties;
- Funding for an organizer to create an umbrella organization of supportive recovery homes.

In 2003, the Common Ground Process was also created by CPHA in collaboration with neighborhood leaders and treatment providers. The process was a tool for promoting positive dialogue, interactions, and accountability among communities and treatment providers. The tool assisted with creating a memorandum of understanding (MOU), or "good neighbor agreement" between the community and providers, and was subsequently utilized by CPHA in garnering support for the supportive recovery housing initiative in Baltimore.

The Baltimore City Drug Court, also aware of the longstanding housing needs of drug offenders, informally advocated for an investigation of supportive housing conditions and the identification of reputable, safe supportive houses in local neighborhoods. The CPHA Director of Drug Treatment and Community Outreach assisted in this process.

In response to a growing need for safe housing, CPHA submitted an application to the Abell Foundation for a grant to fund an organizer and the development of voluntary standards and a peer review process. The Abell Foundation funds non-profit organizations located in Maryland with over 95 percent of their grants awarded to Baltimore metropolitan area organizations.

Through its efforts, the CPHA and partners had successfully created a forum for dialogue among all stakeholders. At the same time, the supportive recovery housing operators demonstrated a desire to be part of the addictions continuum within the community. Some examples include:

- Joining neighborhood associations;
- Modeling for supportive housing residents the role of a good neighbor, e.g., keeping their houses and yards in good order;
- Creating opportunities for neighborhood residents to become involved with the supportive houses; and
- Participating in the Hot Topics forums and the Supportive Housing Task Force with other stakeholders.

Supportive recovery housing residents also played a role in helping break down some of the barriers, stereotypes, and stigma associated with existing supportive houses by volunteering to shovel snow during the winter months, and mowing grass and painting houses in the summer months. By increasing involvement in the community, residents and housing operators helped change how they were perceived by stakeholders.

Bridging the Gap: Setting Standards for Supportive Housing

In 2005, CPHA was awarded an $80,000 Abell Foundation grant that funded an organizer who developed voluntary standards and guidelines for management of supportive recovery housing. Additionally, based on the recommendation of the Task Force, CPHA created the Baltimore Area Association for Supportive Housing (BAASH). BAASH is an association of supportive housing operators who work together to conduct peer reviews of housing programs and monitor supportive recovery housing standards.

The standards do not address day-to-day operations of the supportive recovery homes, but outline basic life safety codes and other standards modeled closely on the State of Maryland's treatment program regulations. The creation and monitoring of these standards served to enhance the overall reputations of supportive recovery homes.

Supportive Housing: Holistically Addressing the Needs of Residents

Because of the sheer volume of people seeking treatment in the City, there is often minimal case management or follow up once an individual completes treatment and moves into a supportive recovery home. Out of necessity, housing operators have taken on the role of case managers, helping residents maintain their recovery. Operators have encouraged residents to seek employment and provided informal assistance to residents in their job search. Many house operators have familiarized themselves with local employment offices, credit bureaus, child welfare offices, and other local services important to residents. Many are also familiar with local case managers and help residents' access services when feasible. Thus, supportive housing operators, through informal networks, are often able to assist with a wide variety of recovery support resources needed by residents. In addition BAASH has successfully utilized the Common Ground process by establishing MOU's with groups such as the Jericho Ex-offender program increasing referrals to BAASH members.

To further the effectiveness of supportive recovery housing, CPHA has provided clinical training focusing on relapse risk identification and relapse prevention. CPHA also coordinated a day-long training that brought together methadone providers and supportive housing operators in a successful effort to break down the barriers for individuals participating in methadone maintenance treatment. CPHA continues to provide or coordinate training on a variety of topics for BAASH and neighborhood stakeholders. Discussion and training topics are determined during monthly BAASH meetings. Examples of training sessions include: "Supportive Housing Operators 101" and "A Legal Framework for Supportive Housing."

Barriers

Funding continues to be a barrier for the supportive recovery housing programs in Baltimore primarily because most operators prefer their autonomy and remain reticent about becoming licensed facilities. Licensure is required for many funding sources. However, 15 - 20 percent of supportive recovery housing operators are licensed half-way house operators. The primary difference between half-way houses and supportive homes are that treatment is customary in half-way houses. Operators who are certified addictions counselors or licensed social workers were more likely to pursue half-way house licensure and can provide counseling services to residents. Some operators believed that licensure would facilitate access to BSAS funding as well as strengthen support for grant applications. To date, however, foundations have provided most of the funding for supportive recovery housing initiatives in the City of Baltimore.

The lack of data on the efficacy of supportive housing is a limitation in receiving additional funding. The City is currently developing a plan for evaluating the supportive recovery housing programs. Lastly, although progress has been made, stigma associated with addictions continues to be a barrier.

> Changing attitudes is a process that takes time. The experience CPHA has had with the supportive recovery housing process is a testament to the fact that attitudes can be changed.

Lessons Learned

By bringing key stakeholders to the table for frank and open discussions, CPHA and its partners have successfully changed perceptions about supportive recovery housing. Supportive housing is an essential element for many individuals completing treatment and in need of safe living environments in which to continue their recovery. Engaging recovery housing operators and residents in the community is critical to overcoming fear and decreasing mistrust of neighborhood residents. Finally, data are needed to substantiate supportive recovery housing as a viable housing alternative, as well as critical to supporting those in recovery.

Summary

The work of CPHA in assisting supportive recovery housing gained credence in the community and is an example of how a community resource can support recovery-oriented systems of care. Though there is still work to be done in the supportive housing community and in the larger system, the work of CPHA on this issue has helped to initiate systems change. Outcomes include:

- Decreased community opposition toward supportive recovery housing in neighborhoods;
- Increased interest and buy-in from supportive recovery housing operators (e.g., membership in BAASH increased from 15 members to nearly 50 members) and neighborhood residents;
- Increased accountability with voluntary standards and submission to peer review inspections that are criteria for membership in BAASH;
- Increased credibility of supportive recovery housing programs and funding opportunities, and community support;
- Increased collaborations, (e.g., among BAASH and Baltimore City Drug Court and the Jericho Ex-offender program) through MOU's resulting also in increased referrals to BAASH members.

The work of CPHA generally reflects several of the elements of recovery-oriented systems of care developed through the National Summit on Recovery. However, there are areas where the convergence between the Association's work and the Summit's elements is particularly marked. They include:

- **Family and other ally involvement** through BAASH family reunification efforts, resident counseling, and regular family visits that help mend damaged relationships with spouses and children.
- **Systems anchored in the community** through the provision of community-based housing. Supportive recovery homes are located within local neighborhoods providing residents with safe housing and access to community services. Community reintegration provides individuals an opportunity to recover and "give back" to the community.
- **Continuity of care** by providing essential recovery support following discharge from treatment and through linkages with available community resources and networks.
- **Strength-based** by building on the natural qualities of the residents, and their family and friends. Additionally, the housing operators (BAASH) demonstrate resilience by modeling successful recovery for their residents.
- **Commitment to peer recovery support** through employing peers as supportive housing operators in supportive recovery homes.
- **Inclusion of the voices and experiences of recovering individuals and their families** by gaining buy-in from stakeholders, including people in recovery (e.g., BAASH), and supportive housing residents and their families/significant others.

CONCLUSION

The four case studies presented in this document reflect innovative strategies for developing recovery-oriented systems of care anchored in diverse communities and targeting a range of populations.

Each organization approached systems-change differently, some as a part of a larger coalition, others as the lead organization creating internal change. Moreover, the motivating factors influencing systems-change varied. For example, Fayette Companies was motivated to develop and pilot the Behavioral Health Recovery Management project because the staff observed that the organization's clinical and business practices were not only ineffective but potentially damaging to the long-term recovery prospects of those they served. The State of Illinois, through the Sheridan Treatment and Re-entry Program, responded to unprecedented recidivism rates that were clearly linked to drug and alcohol use and ineffective approaches to re-entry. White Bison on the other hand, saw that an existing recovery support service, AA, while effective in some cultural settings, was of much more limited value in the Native American cultural context. In response, the Wellbriety Movement was created, integrating key elements of AA and Native American culture. Lastly, CPHA brought together a coalition to provide a critical recovery support service (housing) and community resource. In doing so, they addressed issues of stigma, funding, and housing standards in response to individual and community needs.

Several key themes emerge from each of the case studies. The need for strong leadership was consistently found to be a critical element in successful systems change efforts. Articulating a clear vision and the goals of the systems change process, as well as an effective strategy for communicating them to all parties involved, was also important. Serious consideration must also be given to which key stakeholders from the community or State are included in systems-change planning and implementation. Once the key players are identified, ongoing communication is essential. Evaluation was identified as an important element that should be included from the beginning of the process. Benchmarks, outcomes, and evaluation guidelines must be established at the outset to effectively monitor performance and to demonstrate program/organizational effectiveness to potential funding sources. Finally, providers consistently stated that systems change efforts are far from easy and must be undertaken with an understanding that the process requires a long-term commitment on the part of all stakeholders involved.

In conclusion, the providers stressed that systems change is an effort that must be undertaken to improve the current weaknesses in the systems, thereby providing quality services and maximizing limited resources. The providers believe that efforts towards systems change will ultimately benefit policymakers, advocates, clinicians, the community, and most importantly, the individuals with substance use disorders and their families.

APPENDIX

Several individuals provided invaluable assistance in the development of these case studies and deserve our gratitude for their time and support of this effort. They also deserve to be recognized for implementing systems change efforts that are resulting in recovery-oriented services and systems. The following individuals generously contributed to the content of this document:

Michael Boyle, M.A., President and CEO of Fayette Companies—Behavioral Health Recovery Management Project

Don Coyhis, Founder and President of White Bison, Inc.—The Wellbriety Movement

Pam Rodriguez, M.A., Executive Vice President of TASC, Inc.—Sheridan Drug Treatment Prison and Re-entry Program

Carlos Hardy, M.H.S., Executive Director of NCADD-Maryland Affiliate—The Citizens Planning and Housing Association of Baltimore

REFERENCES

White, W. L., Boyle, M. G., Loveland, D. L. & Corrigan, P. W. (2003). What Is Behavioral Health Recovery Management? A Brief Primer. The Behavioral Health Recovery Management Project, Illinois http://www.bhrm.org/papers/BHRM%20primer.pdf.

White Bison Website. (2007). http://www.whitebison.org/about/philosophy.html.

End Notes

[1] Michael Boyle, et. al. "The Behavioral Health Recovery Management Project: Project Summary and Concept." June 28, 2000. Located online at http://www.bhrm.org/bhrmpsummary.pdf.

[2] "What is Behavioral Health Recovery Management? A Brief Primer." Located online at http://www.bhrm.org/papers/BHRM%20primer.pdf.

[3] Ibid.

[4] Ibid.

[5] Ibid.

[6] Don Coyhis and Richard Simonelli, "Wellbriety-Continuing a Legacy of Resistance – Implementing a Vision for Healing." *Counselor*. August 2006, 7:4. 12.

[7] Ibid., 13.

[8] Ibid.

[9] White Bison, Inc. website located at http://www.whitebison.org/wellbriety_Movement/index.html.

[10] *Counselor*, 12.

[11] White Bison website.

[12] ANCSA.net, Alaska Native Claims Settlement Network located at http://www.ancsa.net/taxonomy

[13] Coyhis and Simonelli, "Rebuilding Native American Communities." *Child Welfare*. March/April 2005, LXXXIV:2. 325.

[14] Ibid.

[15] Ibid.

[16] *Counselor*, 14.

[17] *Child Welfare*, 332.

[18] *Counselor*, 16.

[19] Ibid.

[20] "Governor's Proposal for Department of Corrections Budget Increases Efficiency Through Restructuring, Expands Supervision of Parolees and Re-entry Management," Press release from Governor Rod Blagojevich, February 18, 2004. Located at http://www.idoc.state.il.us/subsections/news/archive/2004/2004-GovProposal ForCorrections.shtml.

[21] Ibid.

[22] Treatment Alternatives for Safe Communities, Inc. (TASC) is an Illinois-based, not-for-profit organization providing behavioral health recovery management services for individuals with substance use and mental health disorders.

[23] TASC, Inc. website located at http://www.tasc.org/preview/corrections.html#rcsp.

[24] Clinical re-entry case management is intensive case management for people leaving prison. TASC case managers provide a referral to treatment, place individuals in treatment, and provide ongoing case management services while individuals are under parole supervision. Clinical re-entry case managers begin meeting with clients prior to their release from prison.

[25] "Supportive Housing in Baltimore City," Task Force Report. March 14, 2005.

In: Recovery-Oriented Systems of Care for Individuals … ISBN: 978-1-62808-648-5
Editor: Jonah Edelman

Chapter 5

RECOVERY-ORIENTED SYSTEMS OF CARE (ROSC) RESOURCE GUIDE*

Melanie Whitter, Donna J. Hillman and Peggie Powers

ACKNOWLEDGMENT

This technical assistance resource guide was prepared for the Substance Abuse and Mental Health Services Administration's (SAMHSA's) Partners for Recovery (PFR) Initiative by Melanie Whitter and Donna J. Hillman of Abt Associates Inc. and Peggie Powers, consultant to Abt Associates Inc. Shannon B. Taitt, M.P.A., served as the Government Project Officer.

NOTE: The authors do not work for the government.

INTRODUCTION

Are you looking for resources on resiliency and recovery-oriented systems of care (ROSC)? Further, have you been reading the headlines concerning national health care reform and wondering how it will impact programs and services within a ROSC? This guide, which contains information from the Substance Abuse and Mental Health Services Administration (SAMHSA), and your colleagues around the country, will assist you with answers to these questions. State and local policy makers responsible for substance use programming, as well as providers of treatment and recovery support services, can look to this guide for information to enhance prevention, treatment, and recovery services as the changes in health care evolve in their communities.

The purpose of this resource guide is to share an overview of ROSC and illustrate how these systems are an integral part of the new health care environment. This guide will align the tenets of health care reform to the benefits, framework, and history of ROSC, and the

* This chapter was released by the Substance Abuse and Mental Health Services Administration, September 2010.

steps for planning and implementing ROSC. Following each section of the guide's narrative, you will find websites to direct you to specific resources that will assist you in conceptualizing and developing ROSC. The resources in this guide include research studies, white papers, conference presentations, manuals, practice guides, check lists, regulations and a number of other documents that have been prepared in response to the need for systems reform.

The establishment of ROSC is a relatively new concept in the substance use disorder field. The structure of ROSC will likely evolve as these systems mature and are evaluated. However, as States and communities are creating and implementing ROSC, they can learn from one another. At the same time that they are developing ROSC, they must also consider the changes that are occurring as a result of health care reform. Some policy makers and providers have begun to assess their community strengths and needs in this regard and formulate ROSC plans that are compatible with the tenets of national health care reform. We hope this resource guide will assist with that process.

One of the most important elements of national health care reform is the expansion of coverage for those with substance use and mental health disorders. The law also requires 'parity' or that group health insurance plans that provide coverage for mental health and substance use disorders be equal to coverage provided for other medical and surgical benefits. These sweeping changes form the foundation for the new health care environment. Ingrained in health care reform is a public health model that supports ROSC through its vision of prevention, screening and early intervention, treatment, and recovery, integrated with primary health care. Complex developments that include new benefit packages and financing strategies, greater use of technology, promotion of evidence-based practices, and the very important linkage with primary care all present opportunities and challenges that will be addressed in months and years to come. For this reason, this resource guide will be a very fluid product. As information on new initiatives and findings becomes available, it will be incorporated into the resource guide to further illuminate this new environment.

The goal of this guide is to arm you with sufficient information to leverage resources that will create the most favorable outcomes for individuals, families and communities.

ROSC in the New Health Care Environment

> "A ROSC is a coordinated network of community-based services and supports that is person-centered and builds on the strengths and resiliencies of individuals, families, and communities to achieve abstinence and improved health, wellness, and quality of life for those with or at risk of alcohol and drug problems.'

The central focus of a ROSC is to create an infrastructure or "system of care' with the resources to effectively address the full range of substance use problems within communities. The specialty substance use disorder field provides the full continuum of care (prevention, early intervention, treatment, continuing care and recovery) in partnership with other disciplines, such as mental health and primary care, in a ROSC. A ROSC encompasses a menu of individualized, person-centered, and strength-based services within a self-defined network. By design, a ROSC provides individuals and families with more options with which to make informed decisions regarding their care. Services are designed to be accessible, welcoming, and easy to navigate. A fundamental value of a ROSC is the involvement of people in recovery, their families, and the community to continually improve access to and quality of services. The table below further illustrates the range of recovery-oriented services that may be offered in a ROSC.

Examples of Recovery-Oriented Activities

	Prevention	Intervention	Treatment	Post-Treatment
Examples of Recovery-Oriented Activities	• Early screening before onset • Collaborate with other systems, e.g., Child welfare, VA. • Stigma reduction activities • Refer to intervention treatment services	• Screening • Early intervention • Pre-treatment • Recovery support services • Outreach services	• Menu of treatment services • Recovery Support services • Alternative services and therapies • Prevention for families and siblings of individuals in treatment	• Continuing care • Recovery support services • Check-ups • Self-monitoring

Traditionally, recovery-oriented services have been viewed as long-term recovery related activities that occur after a formal substance use treatment episode. However, recovery-oriented activities and approaches are also part of the full continuum of care available to persons within a ROSC. Substance use problems are preventable, but left untreated can progress into more serious conditions and can become chronic. A ROSC provides a network of services and supports to address the full spectrum of substance use problems, from harmful use to chronic conditions. Through education, communities are strengthened by recovery-oriented activities that can prevent inappropriate substance use before it occurs. Education also raises awareness about the disease, dispels myths that foster stigma and discrimination, and provides early intervention for those at risk of developing substance use conditions.

A ROSC supports the premise that there are many pathways to recovery. Recovery-oriented activities include providing a menu of traditional treatment services and alternative therapies, including peer recovery coaching, acupuncture, meditation, and music and art therapy. Recovery support services, including employment assistance, child care, care management and housing support, may enhance the engagement of individuals and their families in achieving and sustaining recovery.

The following websites will provide you with background material to assist in understanding recovery-oriented activities and approaches:

- Guiding Principles and Elements of Recovery-Oriented Systems: What do we know from the research? http://pfr.samhsa.gov/docs/Guiding Principles Whitepaper.pdf
- Recovery as an Organizing Concept http://www.facesandvoicesofrecovery.org /pdf/recovery symposium/GLATTCInterviewClark.pdf

- Building Resilience, Wellness and Recovery: A Shift from Acute Care to a Sustained Care Recovery http://www.nattc.org/ Go to Resources & Publications; Type Building Resilience, Wellness and Recovery' in Search bar and press 'Go.'
- Connecticut Department of Mental Health and Addiction Services: Proposed Model for Mental Health Recovery and Recovery-Oriented Services http://www.ct.gov /dmhas/lib/dmhas/recovery/mhmodel.pdf
- The Institute for Research, Education, and Training in Addictions (IRETA) http://www.ireta.org/
- Faces and Voices of Recovery: Guide to Mutual Aid Resources http://www.faces andvoicesofrecovery.org/resources/support/index.html

Like other chronic health conditions, substance use disorders typically require long-term involvement with the health care system and parallel informal networks. Recovery-oriented services and supports include provision of continuing care following treatment, education regarding self-care, regular check-ups and linkage to community resources.

Increasingly, technology is being used in a ROSC to improve access to services through e-therapy, to assist with information sharing, to increase quality and efficiency through use of electronic health records, and to support recovery through social networks. Proficiency with technology will become all the more critical as health care reform is implemented and integration with primary care occurs. A multi-disciplinary workforce is also viewed as critical to delivering quality care in a ROSC. The workforce may include prevention staff, treatment counselors, nurses, doctors, a marriage and family therapist, a psychologist, peer coaches, etc. In a ROSC, organizations are guided by a set of values, goals, elements, core functions, and outcomes to achieve the ROSC's mission. To promote the health of individuals, families and communities, a public health approach is adopted. Substance use disorders are biopsychosocial conditions. These conditions are influenced by various social determinants of health—for example, the social and physical environment, income, education, and life skills. Only by understanding these determinants and applying strategies to influence them can the disease be impacted.

A public health approach focuses on prevention of substance use problems in the general population, and addresses symptoms when they first emerge, rather than when they become acute or chronic. A public health approach also uses data to monitor health problems and evaluate the effectiveness of services, and relies on interdisciplinary methods and partnerships.

The diagram pictured illustrates a ROSC framework that includes the mission, values, goals, system elements, core functions, and outcomes of the systems. The principles of a ROSC and health care are closely aligned—for example, invest in prevention and wellness, expand coverage, guarantee choice, and improve quality of care. A major component of a ROSC is implementing the provisions of health care reform to provide high-quality substance use services. To achieve reform, integration of substance use services will need to occur within primary care settings. Primary care providers will likely require additional education and training on how to screen and intervene with at-risk populations, and on how to refer individuals with more severe conditions to specialty settings. Additionally, specialty providers may be required to establish new partnerships, enhance technology, establish quality improvement systems, expand capacity, recruit and train staff, and work with health insurance plans.

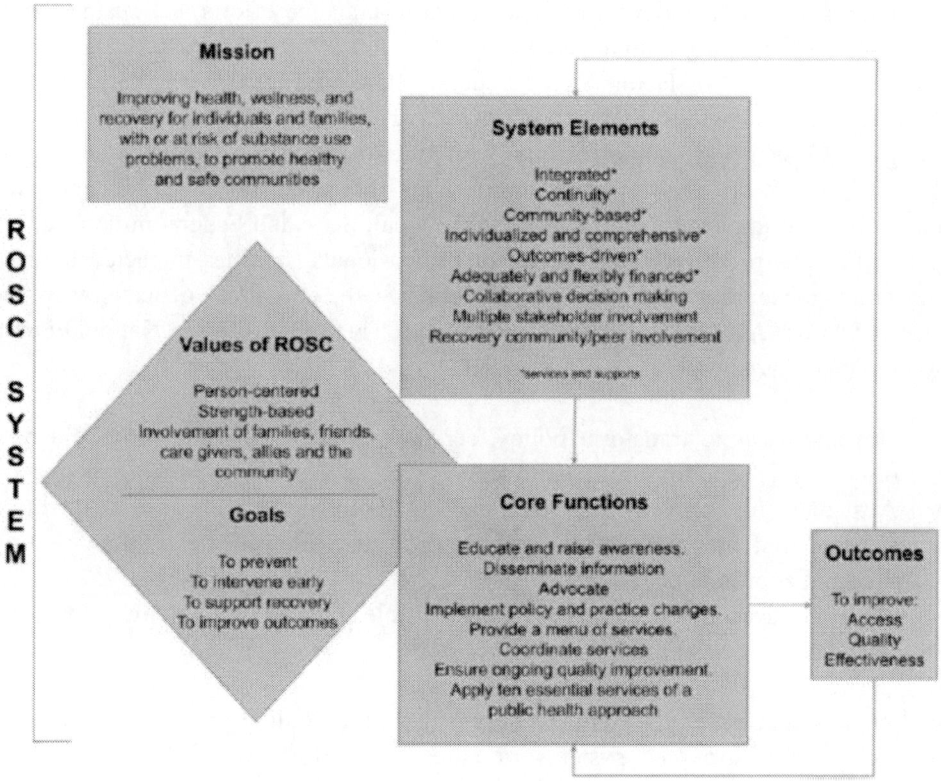

The following websites will provide you with information on the ROSC framework and health care reform:

- Perspectives on Systems Transformation: How Visionary Leaders are Shifting Addiction Treatment Towards a Recovery-Oriented System of Care (ROSC) http://www.attcnetwork.org/regcenters/productdetails.asp?prodID=258&rcID=3
- Coalition for Whole Health: Summary of Recommendations for Including Mental Health and Substance Use Disorder Prevention, Treatment, Rehabilitation, and Recovery in Health Reform http://lac.org/doc library/lac/publications/CWH--Healthcare Reform Recommendations-- summary.pdf
- The Effects of Health Care Reform on Access to, and Funding of, Substance Abuse Services in Maine, Massachusetts, and Vermont http://www.nasadad.org/resource.php?base id=2104
- Vermont Health Care Reform Legislation http://hcr.vermont.gov/legislation

History of ROSC

Implementation of ROSC continues to evolve today, and the passage of national health care reform has opened another potential door in support of ROSC. As more of the public responds to the integration of ROSC within the public health model, there will be additional lessons learned and further development of tools to enhance efforts and sustain health and human services systems at multiple levels.

Thus far, a number of factors at the Federal, State, and local levels have converged to initiate and support the development of ROSC. They include advances in research and technology, release of influential reports (i.e., the Institute of Medicine Quality Chasm Series), growth of the recovery community, an increased focus on collaboration and accountability, and implementation of successful local, State and Federal initiatives. In 2005, key policy makers, prevention and treatment professionals, families impacted by substance use disorders, persons in recovery, and Federal, State, and local officials were brought together at SAMHSA's Center for Substance Abuse Treatment (CSAT) National Summit on Recovery. Their charge was to:

- Develop ideas to transform policy, services, and systems that provide a recovery-oriented response for family members, as well as the persons seeking recovery.
- Articulate guiding principles and measures of recovery that are adaptable across services and programs while supporting system improvements, data sharing, and program coordination.
- Generate ideas that advance ROSC in multiple settings and systems, and for specific populations.

Participants successfully reached a consensus on the guiding principles of recovery and elements of recovery-oriented systems of care. This effort provided the framework for additional discussions and engagement by persons in communities across the country.

Opportunities for ROSC abound, as systems are integrated and transformed through coordination, communication, and linkage. SAMHSA and the substance use disorder field have begun to conceptualize the magnitude of this paradigm shift. The history of ROSC continues to be written as the focus of health care reform broadly encompasses the continuum of care for substance use disorders.

In order to learn more about the guiding principles of recovery and the early conceptual work done to define the systems elements of a ROSC, refer to the following website:

- National Summit on Recovery: Conference Report http://pfr.samhsa.gov/ Enter 'National Summit on Recovery' in the Search bar.

Additional resources associated with the history of ROSC, including reports, research briefs, monographs, training manuals, and presentations can be found at:

- The Institute for Research, Education, and Training in Addictions (IRETA) http://www.ireta.org/

RECOVERY SUPPORT SERVICES (RSS)

Each of the partners in a ROSC can play a role in the provision of recovery support services. When RSS are provided across the continuum of care, they support resiliency, open doors to service access and engagement, and support long-term recovery. Person-centered supports bolster successful individual and family outcomes.

Recovery support services are non-clinical services that assist individuals and families working towards recovery from substance use disorders. They incorporate a full range of social, legal, and other resources that facilitate recovery and wellness to reduce or eliminate environmental or personal barriers to recovery. RSS include social supports, linkage to and coordination among allied service providers, and other resources to improve quality of life for people in and seeking recovery and their families. RSS are provided by professionals and peers and are delivered through a variety of community and faith-based groups, treatment providers, and RSS providers. Provision of RSS is based upon the needs in a person's individualized recovery plan.

While typically viewed as available post-treatment, recovery support services within the construct of ROSC can be offered before, during, or even in lieu of treatment. This approach and its supports are inclusive of pre-treatment, as well as promotion of resiliency in prevention and early or brief interventions. These are tenets that also form the basis of a public health model and are aligned with the principles of health care reform.

Child care and transportation are two of the most commonly recognized support services, but States and providers must leverage other systems to assemble a broader menu of resources as they implement ROSC. By looking across the entire continuum and addressing supports specific to the individual, ROSC can identify a myriad of resources that may be used to foster recovery. Housing, life skills training, help with employment readiness, and legal consultation are examples of support that may be beyond what a ROSC currently provides, but which are often important to supporting recovery. Wellness checks, which support healthy lifestyles, are currently used in primary care settings for persons who have chronic conditions such as diabetes or heart disease. This same practice can be replicated for persons with substance use disorders.

In addition to tangible resources like housing and transportation, there is a human element that is equally valuable in the provision of RSS. A peer mentor or recovery coach can be very effective in providing motivation and support as an individual seeks a recovery lifestyle. When an established frame of reference reflects their own recovery process, peer mentors and recovery coaches are valuable assets in recovery support. They can bring significant interpersonal skills to their work with individuals engaged in or contemplating recovery. As a ROSC moves further into the implementation phase, peer-driven supports will become a part of the fabric of recovery that cannot be replicated by other resources.

Beyond the RSS functions that often require certification, States will be challenged to develop core competencies or minimal guidelines for persons and organizations who deliver these services. Although health care reform and parity legislation will enable some service billing through insurance carriers for RSS, they may have more-stringent requirements related to service delivery for RSS than for conventional medical treatment. When peer-driven services are initiated, consideration should be given to a reasonable match of gender, education, ethnicity and recovery philosophy, as well as defined core competencies.

As a ROSC implements RSS, a few key steps can guide the process:

- Secure a broad range of supports through leverage with all partner systems.
- Focus on the specific needs of the individuals and families.
- Engage peer recovery coaches who have a personal recovery focus.

- Define competency guidelines. (Competency guidelines should reflect requirements of third- party insurance carriers if possible.)

Resources found below can assist States and providers to achieve these steps.

- An RCSP Conference Report: Emerging Peer Recovery Support Services and Indicators of Quality http://www.facesandvoicesofrecovery.org/pdf/Publications /2006-09 RCSP Report.pdf
- Ethical Guidelines for the Delivery of Peer-based Recovery Support Services http://www.bhrm.org/recoverysupport/EthicsPaperFinal6-8-07.pdf
- Manual for Recovery Coaching and Personal Recovery Plan http://www.bhrm.org Select 'Clinical Guidelines'; select 'Addiction Guidelines; scroll down to 'Recovery Coach and Recovery Planning Manual
- Center for Substance Abuse Treatment: What are Peer Recovery Support Services http://store.samhsa.gov/product/SMA09-4454
- Recovery Coach Training Manual http://www.nattc.org/resPubs/changeBook.html
- Financing Recovery Support Services: Review and Analysis of Funding Recovery Support Services and Policy Recommendations http://pfr.samhsa.gov/docs/RSS financing report.pdf
- Vermont Substance Abuse Recovery - provides access to the Recovery Centers Website; Friends of Recovery-Vermont (consumer/advocacy network); and the Vermont Peer Resources Guide http://healthvermont.gov/adap/recovery /Recovery.aspx

ROLE OF RECOVERY MANAGEMENT

Within the framework of a ROSC, recovery management provides treatment and recovery supports to individuals with severe substance use disorders. This targeted approach to a specific population differs from the overarching role of a ROSC. As has been described, a ROSC serves those with or at risk for substance use problems. The persons served within a ROSC encompass the general population, at-risk populations, harmful users of alcohol and drugs, those with dependence, and those with chronic dependence.

Recovery management is often described as typifying the shift from an acute care model, which treats medical conditions in an intensive short-term manner, to a chronic care approach reflecting a service commitment to long-term supports and wellness. A ROSC provides a full spectrum of services based on individual need. These may include early intervention service (i.e., Screening, Brief Intervention and Referral to Treatment), acute care services (i.e., medically managed detoxification), and chronic care services (i.e., continuing care followed by recovery checkups, otherwise known as Recovery Management).

The public health community has long practiced recovery management when treating chronic diseases such as diabetes, asthma, and hypertension. While public health care providers may use different terminology, recovery management is a tool embedded in their approach to practice. Public health principles address health promotion through comprehensive prevention strategies, screening, early intervention, treatment, and reinforcement of healthy lifestyles. Sound familiar? This model is also found in ROSC, and one that is the cornerstone of the new health care environment.

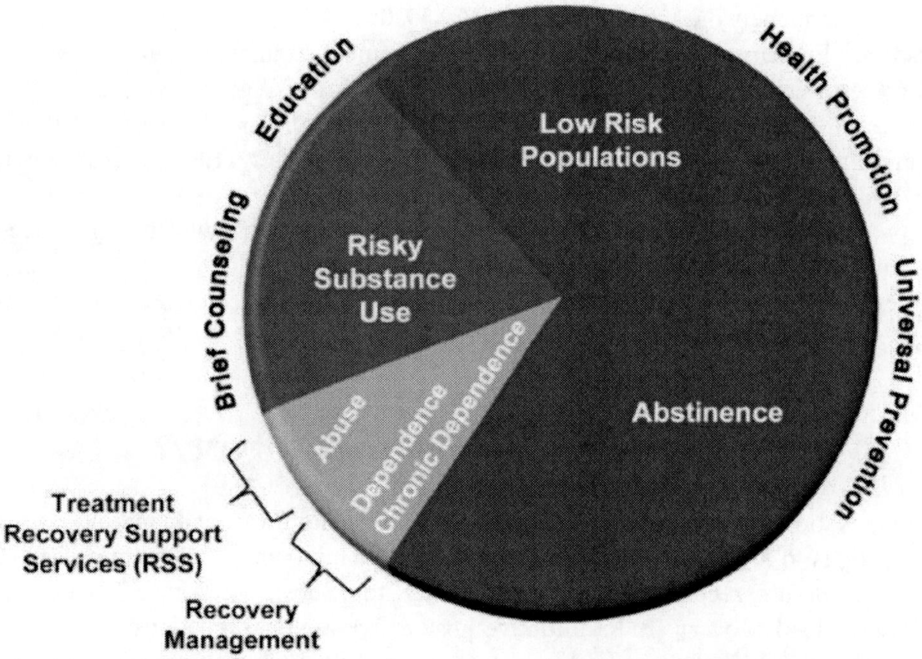

Recovery Management (RM)
Recovery Management engages individuals with chronic substance use conditions and assists the person in managing efforts to achieve long-term recovery.

Activities: Establish assertive engagement processes; conduct strength-based assessments; provide recovery-focused and person-centered treatment/recovery support services; train clients on self-care; provide post-treatment check-ups; use community resources to support sustained recovery

Recovery-Oriented Systems of Care (ROSC)
ROSC encompass the general population, at-risk populations, harmful users of alcohol and drugs, those with dependence, and those with chronic dependence.

Functions: Inform, educate and empower individuals and communities; provide prevention, early intervention, treatment and recovery services; recommend/implement policy and practice changes; mobilize community partnerships; evaluate services for ongoing systems improvement

Recovery management engages individuals with chronic substance use conditions and assists the person in managing efforts to achieve long-term recovery. Individuals and their families are empowered to seek supports specific to meet the needs of the person. There is no formula or set of rote practices that serve everyone. Different persons require different resources. It is the role of recovery management to coordinate access to resources and foster engagement. ROSC coordinate the layers of multiple systems that can produce those resources. As a result of the collaborative work done by a ROSC, these systems—including criminal justice, education, child welfare, and primary care—can provide the supports necessary to sustain recovery management activities.

To learn more about the role of recovery management within ROSC, please access the following websites:

- Implementing Recovery Management Part 1: The Organizing Concept http://www.attcnetwork.org/learn/topics/rosc/docs/AddicMsgVol.11,Issue4NEW.pdf
- Implementing Recovery Management Part 2: Making the Philosophical Shift http://www.attcnetwork.org/userfiles/file/Vol.%2011,%20Issue%205%20NEW.pdf
- Frontline Implementation of Recovery Management Principles http://www.faces andvoicesofrecovery.org/pdf/recovery symposium/GLATTCInterviewBoyle.pdf
- Recovery Management & Recovery-Oriented Systems of Care: Scientific Rationale & Promising Practices http://www.attcnetwork.org/REGCENTERS/generalContent.asp?rcid=3&content=STCUSTOM1
- Recovery Management in Communities of Color http://www.nattc.org/recovery resourc/docs/RecMgmt.pdf
- Implementing Recovery Management Part 3: Recovery Coaching Pays Dividends http://www.nattc.org/userfiles/file/Vol.%2011,%20Issue%206%20NEW(1).pdf

What Is Happening Around the Country?

At the 2005 National Summit on Recovery, a recommendation was made to hold a series of regional meetings to assist States and communities in planning and implementing ROSC. Following the Summit's recommendation, the Center for Substance Abuse Treatment's (CSAT's) Partners for Recovery (PFR) Initiative hosted five regional meetings in 2007 and early 2008 to support ROSC planning and implementation at the State and community levels. Teams from 49 States, the District of Columbia, and Puerto Rico participated.

At that time, the stages of ROSC implementation across the country ranged from active planning and systemic re-engineering to very preliminary consideration of the ROSC concept. Of those States attending the regional meetings, 10 percent (5 States) were engaged in active planning and implementation of ROSC, 35 percent (18 States) were implementing system elements and had begun planning for ROSC, 43 percent (22 States) had implemented one or more system elements, and 12 percent (6 States) were considering implementing ROSC.

As a part of the work done during the regional meetings, State teams were asked to envision a ROSC that reflected their own locale's unique environment, inclusive of challenges and creative solutions to work within existing systems. They were then asked to develop an action plan to identify steps that have been taken, and what steps need to be taken to facilitate implementation of ROSC.

After the regional meetings, a number of States moved forward in implementing a recovery-oriented framework. These states have cultivated partnerships with the medical community, among other systems, and are poised to further implement the tenets of health care reform in their alcohol and drug programming. Following are examples of State ROSC activities:

California

In 2006, the California Department of Alcohol and Drug Programs (CADP) began a multi-year process to support system evolution from an acute care model to one of chronic care. Established by CADP, the Continuum of Services System Re-Engineering Task Force have led this effort through engagement of stakeholders, development of core principles and goals, and creation of a website containing their presentations, findings, and other materials that reflect the principles of ROSC. As with most States, resources have diminished, but California remains committed to supporting a client- centered chronic care system that is inclusive of prevention, treatment, and recovery.

North Carolina

A task force, convened at the direction of the North Carolina General Assembly and led by the North Carolina Institute of Medicine, has steered the State's efforts to plan and implement ROSC. In addressing the full continuum of care, the task force published a comprehensive report that provided significant recommendations for a system redesign that reflects the principles of ROSC. Their work was taken a step further by the legislature when this model was embedded in State statutes. Today, much of the activity centers around training and a public campaign called 'Recovery North Carolina.' The campaign has successfully engaged an advisory board, as well as volunteers and community members throughout the State.

North Carolina also redirected funds through an RFP process to allow provider flexibility in establishing services to support ROSC. The challenges that remain in North Carolina are primarily lack of funding and lack of a data system to support the success of evidence-based practices.

Vermont

Prior to the regional meetings, Vermont had begun to construct a framework for recovery activities, called Friends of Recovery – VT. Following the CSAT-sponsored meetings, and with technical assistance from their ATTC, Vermont began to formalize ROSC through the establishment of a strategic plan and mission statement. The plan ensured that all stakeholders understood the principles and concept of ROSC. In addition, a State initiative, the Vermont Blueprint for Health, provided a statewide structure and a vehicle to more effectively manage chronic diseases using a public health model in tandem with ROSC. With the strategic plan, mission, and Friends of Recovery – VT in place, the State initiated a series of provider trainings with the assistance of NIATx. Incentives planning grants and monthly learning calls have further bolstered Vermont's efforts to implement ROSC.

Steps have been taken to ensure that the prevention community is part of the overall continuum, and that a strong family focus and resiliency are integral to ROSC. Vermont has termed their systems change approach a Resiliency and Recovery-Oriented Systems of Care (RROSC). Vermont has instituted telephone recovery checkups, fostered peer support, and strengthened an integrated approach to RROSC.

The websites below will provide you with additional information on these and other initiatives that are underway across the country.

- National Summary of CSAT's Regional Recovery Meetings http://pfr.samhsa.gov /recovery.html
- A Recovery Revolution in Philadelphia http://www.ireta.org Enter the title in the Search bar and press 'Go.'
- Continuum of Services System Re-Engineering Report, September 24, 2008 http://www.adp.cahwnet.gov/COSSR
- Vermont Blueprint for Health http://hcr.vermont.gov/blueprint for health
- Building a Recovery-Oriented System of Care: A Report of the NCIOM Task Force on Substance Abuse Services, January, 2009. http://www.nciom.org/wp-content /uploads/NCIOM/projects/substance abuse/chapters/FullReport.pdf

The following three documents can be found at: http://pfr.samhsa.gov/rosc.html

- Access to Recovery (ATR) Approaches to Recovery-Oriented Systems of Care: Three Case Studies
- Provider Approaches to Recovery-Oriented Systems of Care: Four Case Studies
- Approaches to Recovery-Oriented Systems of Care at the State and Local Levels: Three Case Studies

Planning and Implementation Steps

Creating a ROSC requires thoughtful and strategic planning, particularly as policymakers, providers, the recovery community, and the general public negotiate systems changes that involve the integration of substance use services within the general health care system. This evolution is ongoing, so be mindful of its implications as you plan and implement ROSC within your State or community. Identifying where you are in the ROSC planning and implementation process, while being cognizant of the new health care environment, will guide you in determining priorities and next steps.

The diagram below reflects the steps that are integral to establishing a systems change process. Each will be further described in this resource guide.

A **Readiness Assessment** should examine your willingness and ability to establish a platform for a ROSC. A coalition of stakeholders should be engaged to consider important questions that examine the level of commitment and feasibility for the effort. That dialogue may prompt divergent opinions before you reach a consensus. However, that is to be expected, given the time and effort needed to construct a functional ROSC. A facilitator with no vested interested in the outcome can play a key role in keeping the discussion moving and maintaining a record of the proceedings.

In assessing readiness, there are core questions that, when answered, will drive the consideration for systems change. The following table can be used to frame that discussion.

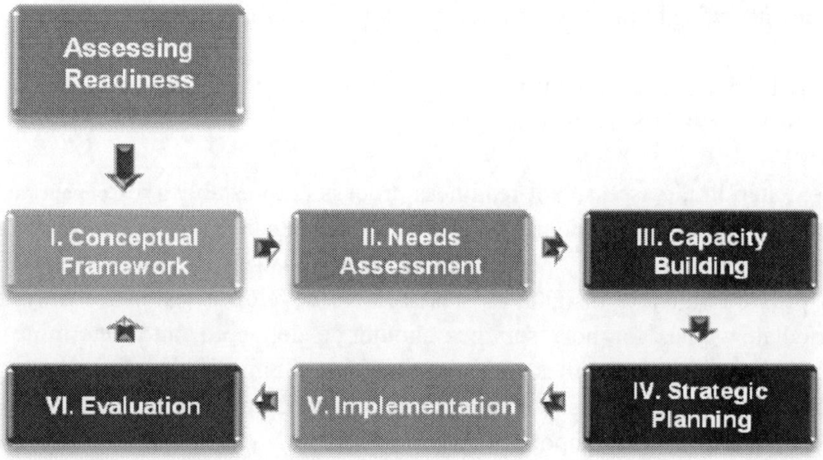

Assessing Readiness: Core Considerations in Preparing for Change

Initial Consideration	Further Considerations
1. Can you build a compelling case for change?	• What is the compelling case for creating a ROSC at this time? • What problems will be solved? • What value will be added to the system? • What currently is being done in your community to address substance use problems and disorders? • How effective are the current interventions? • Will change be better than business as usual?
2. Are the anticipated results compelling enough to initiate and sustain the change process?	• What are the desired results from adopting a ROSC? • Results for your community? • Results for families and involved others? • Results for persons in or seeking recovery? • By when do you expect to see these results? • What measures will you use to assess progress and impact?
3. Are the essential stakeholders willing and able to commit to and champion ROSC over time?	• Who will be the *sponsors* and advocates of a ROSC change initiative in your community? • Are the sponsors able to initiate and sustain support for the process?
4. Are the potential benefits of change, and the consequences of "business as usual,' sufficient for community stakeholders to support ROSC implementation?	• What are the consequences of continuing systems as they currently exist? • For the key stakeholders, what are the rewards associated with supporting and participating in the ROSC initiative? • What are their incentives for sustained engagement?
5. Are there sufficient systems and resources in your community to support implementation of ROSC?	• How much will it cost to adopt a ROSC? • Are stakeholders willing and able to assure the systems and resources necessary to fully sustain a ROSC over time?

You may also wish to use the resource below to further aid in the assessment process.

- Community Readiness Survey http://www.ncspfsig.org/Project Docs/Community%20Readiness%20Survey2.doc

The next step in the assessment readiness process is to establish a **Conceptual Framework**. Use of focus groups and key participant interviews can ensure input from a broad spectrum of the community. Participation by persons in recovery, as well as family members and other allies, can provide valuable insights as stakeholders develop a vision for a system of care, clearly articulate values for how services should be delivered, and determine the desired outcomes for individuals, families and communities. Some of the questions posed to the stakeholder group during the assessment readiness exercise may help structure the conceptual framework. In addition, other important questions are:

- What is your definition of recovery?
- What should a ROSC look like in your community?
- Why is a change needed?
- What outcomes do you hope to achieve through a ROSC?

A discussion and consideration of these issues should result in a common vision, and in common values, system elements, outcomes, and definitions. Without general agreement on the conceptual framework for the ROSC, the process cannot successfully move forward. Below are additional resources to inform your dialogue when developing a conceptual framework.

- Connecticut Recovery Core Value http://www.ct.gov/dmhas/cwp/view.asp?a=2901&q=335078
- Overarching Tenets of the Recovery Initiative http://www.ct.gov/dmhas/LIB/dmhas/Recovery/tenets.pdf
- A Recovery Revolution in Philadelphia http://www.ireta.org/ Enter the title in the Search bar and press 'Go.'

Completion of a **Needs Assessment** is another key step in developing an informed ROSC plan. Stakeholders must understand the extent of substance use problems, the populations affected, gaps in services and supports, and services and systems that require quality improvements. This information will allow you to target and maximize resources. Identifying community and organizational strengths is equally important, as they provide a strong foundation upon which to build. This identification can strengthen discussion among ROSC partners, and provide a path for support in your implementation plan. Stakeholders should also examine policies and practices to assess their alignment with ROSC elements, in order to determine what changes are required to structure a functional ROSC.

- Assessment Primer: Analyzing the Community, Identifying Problems, and Setting Goals http://www.cadca.org/resources/detail/assessment-primer
- Yale Program for Community Health and Recovery: Recovery Self-Assessment (Provider Version) http://www.yale.edu/prch/tools/rec selfassessment.html

The needs assessment process has identified the strengths as well as gaps in services within the current systems. It should now be translated into a plan to enhance the capacity of your system where needed. ***Capacity Building*** is an integral part of successful systems change implementation. Does your ROSC have capacity at all levels, the staff or volunteer level, the organizational level, the broader systems level?

Each systems element should reflect a comprehensive, person-centered, and individualized approach to service provision. It is understandable that all systems may not initially align with this operational philosophy, but it's important to determine what your capacity needs are so that they can be addressed. In addition to workforce capacity, technology and other resources should be considered. For further information on capacity building, see the resources below.

- Capacity Primer: Building Membership, Structure and Leadership http://www.cadca.org/files/CapacityPrimer-07-2009.pdf
- National Certified Recovery Specialist http://www.iaodapca.org/certifications/ncrs/
- Maintaining Abstinence Program: A Curriculum for Families in Recovery http://www.ireta.org/ireta main/recoveryCD/MAPSFamiliesinRecovery-Stages-of-Recovery.pdf
- Pennsylvania OMHSAS: Strategies for Promoting Recovery and Resilience and Implementing Evidence-Based Practices http://www.cmsu.org/recoverydocument.pdf
- Executive Leadership Guidelines for Developing a Behavioral Electronic Health Record System Technology Plan http://www.ndiic.com/documents/Developing %20an%20Electronic%20BH%20Tech%20Plan %2001-27-2010.pdf
- State HIE Resources http://statehieresources.org/state-plans/

The next step in ROSC planning and implementation is development of a ***Strategic Planning Process***. After you have assembled a planning team that represents stakeholder interests, articulated a vision, conducted a needs assessment, and constructed a capacity building plan, it's time to develop a strategic plan including specific ROSC goals. A critical step at this juncture is, once again, to ensure sufficient community representation, inclusive of individuals in recovery, family members and other allies.

Following that, the planning team should be charged with identifying measureable objectives for each goal, as well as strategies to support achievement of each goal. Other tasks that should be completed in order to reinforce a strategic planning process are:

- Developing action steps,
- Identifying timelines and parties responsible for completing each strategy,
- Creating a resource plan, and
- Documenting the entire plan.

To guide you further during the strategic planning process, refer to the information below.

- Planning Primer: Developing a Theory of Change, Logic Models, and Strategic Action Plans http://www.actmissouri.org/PDF%20Files/Planning.pdf

- Creating a Strategic Plan http://www.ncspfsig.org/Project Docs/Creating%20A%20 Strategic%20Plan How%20To%20G uide.pdf
- Getting to Outcomes: 10 Steps for Achieving Results-based Accountability http://www.rand.org/pubs/technical reports/2007/RAND TR101.2.pdf
- Getting to Outcomes 2004: Promoting Accountability Through Methods and Tools for Planning, Implementation, and Evaluation http://www.rand.org/pubs/technical reports/2004/RAND TR101.pdf

Now that the planning is well underway, it's time to begin assembling the resources for **Implementation**. Engagement of the community at large, as well as individuals in recovery, their families, and other allied members, will strengthen efforts to identify and garner resources for a ROSC. Implementation of ROSC will require changes to a number of institutional practices and processes. Trying to affect change in multiple levels of systems that interact with other multiple levels of systems can be overwhelming. You may initially focus on workforce development, financing, policy enhancement, technology changes to support data tracking and billing, or one of many other topics that will come into play when putting your plan into practice. Due to the complexity and challenges inherent in a major systems change, it may be wise to implement ROSC incrementally.

To further inform your implementation efforts, see the resources listed below.

- Implementation Primer: Putting Your Plan into Action http://www.cadca.org /resources/detail/implementation-primer
- Implementing a Statewide Recovery-Oriented System of Care: From Concept to Reality http://www.ct.gov/dmhas/LIB/dmhas/presentations/2.6.05.pdf
- Connecticut Department of Mental Health and Addiction Services: Proposed Model of Mental Health Recovery and Recovery-Oriented Services: http://www.ct.gov/ dmhas/lib/dmhas/recovery/mhmodel.pdf
- Cultural Competence Primer: Incorporating Cultural Competence into Your Comprehensive Plan http://www.cadca.org/files/cultural competence jan09.pdf
- Connecticut DMHAS. Practice Guidelines for Recovery-Oriented Care for Mental Health and Substance Use Conditions http://www.ct.gov/dmhas/lib/dmhas/recovery /practiceguidelines2.pdf
- Connecticut Implementation of Person-Centered Care http://www.ct.gov /dmhas/LIB/dmhas/Recovery/personcentered.pdf
- California Access to Recovery (CARE) Recovery Support Services Screening and Assessment Tool http://www.californiacares4youth.com/downloads/RSS%20 screening%20and%20assessment% 20tool.pdf
- Practice Guidelines for Recovery-Oriented Behavioral Health Care http://www.ct.gov/dmhas/LIB/dmhas/publications/practiceguidelines.pdf
- Recovery Advocacy Toolkit: Resource Guide http://www.facesandvoicesof recovery.org/publications/advocacy toolkit/resources.php
- Peer/Recovery Support Specialists within Behavioral Health Agencies: Desktop Guide http://www.azdhs.gov/bhs/guidance/peer.pdf

As States and communities move toward implementation of ROSC, *Financing* may become a primary concern. However, broad consideration must be given to all viable funding sources to encourage creative and flexible financing. An initial review of funding resources may focus on Medicaid and the Substance Abuse Prevention and Treatment Block Grant (SAPT BG), but other streams may be leveraged when States are able to braid dollars and access funding from multiple systems. There is great diversity across the country regarding financing of systems of care, and there is not one funding solution that will adequately meet the needs of every community. The key is sufficient flexibility to achieve the best outcomes for individuals, families, and communities.

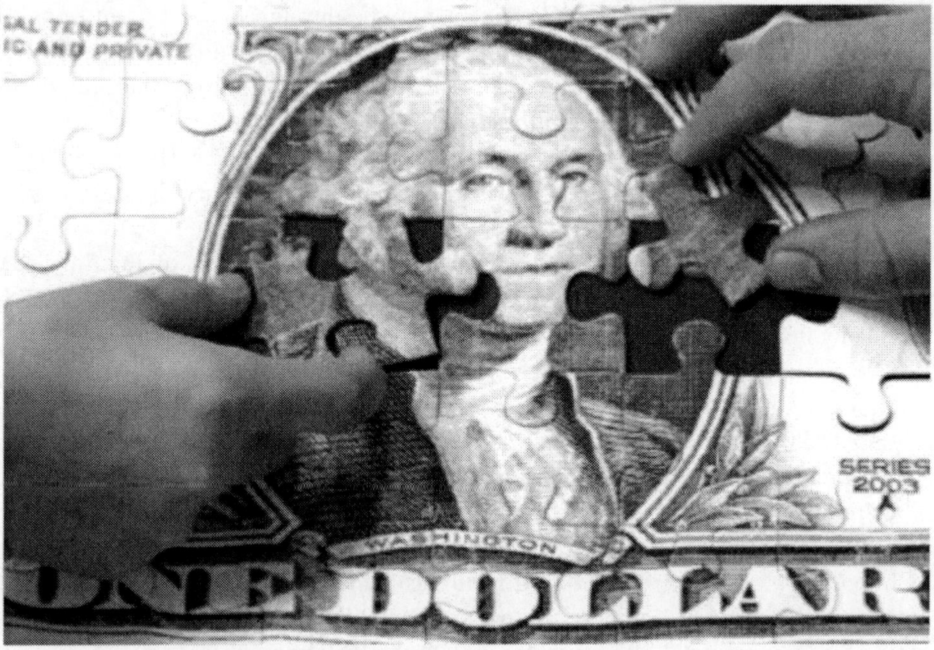

Flexible funding will enable a ROSC to offer individualized and comprehensive services for each person in a manner that best meets their needs. Funding tied to specific program models and approaches that are 'one size fits all' is inconsistent with the person-centered focus of a ROSC. A ROSC that exercises creative financing strategies to offer an array of services tailored to an individual's needs will encourage more successful outcomes. Offering financial incentives to offset systems improvement costs and providing start-up funds to initiate systems change are successful strategies that have been used in States and localities.

While States have historically relied on Medicaid, the SAPT BG, and State general revenue dollars to fund prevention, treatment, and recovery services, those who are planning and implementing ROSC are also accessing resources provided through other systems. Changes resulting from implementation of parity and national health care reform initiatives will open additional doors to service provision.

Some States have already forged a successful collaboration with the justice system, at both the local and Federal levels, to garner funding support for ROSC services. The education community and its prevention resources provide another avenue to enhance ROSC activities and funding. Local environmental strategies shape school prevention initiatives that are broadly supported and funded.

Partnering with school systems ensures the inclusion of prevention as a part of ROSC. Seeking support and building a ROSC framework with multiple partners will bolster resources to sustain the most comprehensive system.

Financing opportunities may also be available from the private sector. As systems collaborate and identify common goals and activities supporting ROSC on a local level, foundation grants and private partner donations can be accessed to fund specific services. This can be achieved by designing a flexible system that satisfies the requirements of the funder while meeting the specific needs of individuals and families.

Another source of financing ROSC changes may be through Federal grant opportunities. An ROSC may secure 'seed money' through grant awards to begin or further progress its systems changes. Once those innovations are realized, cost offsets from the previous system structure may be realized and applied to the ROSC operation.

As you review the resources below, keep in mind that flexible financing can better position your ROSC to meet the unique needs of persons or families seeking services.

- Financing Recovery Support Services: Review and Analysis of Funding Recovery Support Services and Policy Recommendations http://pfr.samhsa.gov/docs/RSS financing report.pdf
- The Effects of Health Care Reform on Access to and Funding of Substance Abuse Services in Maine, Massachusetts, and Vermont http://nasadad.org/resources /Final%20revisions%20HCR%20508%20compliant.pdf
- Sustainability Primer: Fostering Long-Term Change to Create Drug-Free Communities http://www.cadca.org/resources/detail/sustainability-primer
- CMS Letter to State Medicaid Directors on Funding Peer Support Services http://www.cms.hhs.gov/SMDL/downloads/SMD081507A.pdf
- Virginia Recovery Support Demonstration Model http://www.dbhds.virginia.gov /SASC/documents/VARecoverySupportModelRFP.pdf
- Improving Public Addiction Treatment through Performance Contracting: The Delaware Experiment http://www.ncbi.nlm.nih.gov/pmc/articles/PMC2736056/
- Connecticut DMHAS General Assistance Recovery Support Program (GA RSP) http://www.ct.gov/dmhas/cwp/view.asp?a=2900&q=334750

Having the necessary *Policies and Regulations* in place is critical to successful implementation of a ROSC. A thorough inventory of existing policies and regulations will determine which require amendment or modification. This process should also include identification and subsequent development of new policies and regulations that further support the framework for ROSC implementation and ongoing operation. A successful ROSC is made up of multiple stakeholders, representing multiple systems. Thus, the inventory must include a broad range of policies and regulations. These policies exist at the State level and local provider level, and will further unfold at the Federal level as national health care reform is realized.

Within the inventory will be State statutes. Significant changes may be required at the State level to ensure that enabling legislation is in place that reflects the fundamentals of ROSC. In addition to statutes related to the functions of the Single State Agencies (SSA) for Alcohol and other Drugs, language embedded in criminal justice statutes, primary health care statutes and child welfare may require amendment. Following statutory changes, States will develop or amend their Administrative Rules, and issue policy guidelines and interpretations to reflect ROSC fundamentals. Providers and other ROSC partners must also incorporate ROSC-related policies and procedures into their operational directives at the local level.

In order to fund a portion of ROSC services through Medicaid, State Medicaid Plans may require amendment and approval by the Federal Centers for Medicare and Medicaid Services. As national health care reforms crystallize, additional policies and regulations will need to be developed at multiple levels within a ROSC.

The breadth in policy and regulatory changes required to implement a ROSC may seem daunting. But once again, an incremental approach and prioritization of steps to implementation will enable States and providers to move forward in establishing a comprehensive ROSC.

Below are resources to assist States and providers in developing guidelines, policies, and procedures to structure a ROSC.

- Policy Statement #33 - Individualized Recovery Planning http://www.ct.gov/dmhas /cwp/view.asp?a=2907&q=334664
- Michigan DCHODCP Treatment Policy No. 08: Substance Abuse Case Management Program Requirements http://www.michigan.gov/documents/mdch/TA Treatment 03 Case Management Services 17 5208 7.doc
- Michigan DCHODCP Treatment Technical Advisory No. 07: Peer Recovery/ Recovery Support Services http://www.michigan.gov/documents/mdch /TA-T-07 Peer Recovery-Recovery Support 230852 7.pdf
- OMHAS Resilience and Recovery Policy Statement
- http://www.oregon.gov/DHS/addiction/publications/recovery-resil-policy.pdf

Evaluation is integral to a systems change process. It can promote sustainability of effective policies, programs, and practices. It can inform funding decisions, guide clinicians and other service providers when they are working with patients, assist in patient decision making, and educate peers. Evaluation approaches typically look at the processes as well as the outcomes, ranging from short- to long-term goals and objectives.

As component partners within a ROSC begin to forge their resources through collaboration, it is important to consider data collection. Without a mechanism to collect administrative data, it may be difficult to make assumptions concerning performance improvements. Surveys, focus groups, and key informant interviews are also evaluation tools that can be used to strengthen evaluation findings. Stakeholder partners should be encouraged to provide input into the development of these tools in order to increase commitment, broaden their knowledge of the process, and increase the practicality of the evaluation findings. Through ongoing data collection and establishing performance measures you can capture meaningful and immediate response to your ROSC transformation activities.

An effective evaluation systemically tells us:

- How well does the planning process reflect the identified needs, priorities and resources?
- What is implemented—what programs, strategies, activities—and by whom?
- What can we say about 'implementation fidelity'?
- What changes were made along the way and why?

- Where are the successes?
- Where are needed improvements?

Thus far, little evaluation has been conducted on ROSC. This dearth of information highlights the importance of evaluating your recovery-oriented system to improvement them and to more effectively serve your community. Process improvement models are valuable resources to assist you with enhancing your change processes and outcomes. They offer practical approaches to guide and test your work in real-life settings for the purpose of continuous quality improvement.

For information pertaining to evaluation activity, see the resources below.

- Institute for Healthcare Improvement: http://www.ihi.org/IHI/Topics/Improvement /ImprovementMethods/HowToImprove/
- The Network for the Improvement of Addiction Treatment (NIATx): http://www.niatx.net/Content/ContentPage.aspx?PNID=1&NID=7
- CDC Framework for Program Evaluation: http://www.cdc.gov/eval/framework.htm
- Connecticut DMHAS Recovery Self-Assessment: Executive Summary: http://www.ct.gov/dmhas/lib/dmhas/recovery/rsasummary.pdf

Additional ROSC Resources

- Is Your Drug Court Fit for Recovery? A Recovery Check-up http://www.facesandvoicesofrecovery.org/pdf/drug court check list.pdf
- A Conceptual Bridge Between the Mental Health and Addiction Fields http://www.williamwhitepapers.com/pr/2006SystemsTransformation.pdf
- The Recovery Revolution: Will it include children, adolescents, and transition age youth http://www.facesandvoicesofrecovery.org/pdf/White/ChildAdolescents.pdf
- CDC. Principles of Community Engagement http://www.cdc.gov/phppo/pce/
- Guiding Principles and Elements of Recovery-Oriented Systems: What do we know from the research? http://pfr.samhsa.gov/docs/Guiding Principles Whitepaper.pdf

Additional Health Care Reform Resources

- Kaiser Daily Health Policy Daily Reports http://www.kaiserhealthnews.org /Topics/Reform.aspx
- US Department of Health and Human Services, Substance Abuse and Mental Health Services Administration (SAMHSA) Health System Reform: A Framework for Discussion http://www.samhsa.gov/Healthreform/index.aspx
- Trust for America's Health: Prevention and Wellness in Health Care Reform resources http://healthyamericans.org/health-reform/
- National Health Care Reform http://lac.org/index.php/lac/national healthcare reform

- Benefit Design and the Delivery of Care (equitable & full coverage; access) http://lac.org/doc library/lac/publications/CWH--Benefit Design and the Delivery%20of Care.pdf
- Reforming the Health Care Delivery System (workforce development, training all health professionals in MH and SA issues, medical home model, ensuring that MH & SA professionals are included and prioritized in any broader workforce development efforts) http://lac.org/doc library/lac/publications/CWH-- Reforming the Healthcare Delivery System.pdf
- Wellness Promotion and Chronic Disease Prevention Initiatives http://lac.org/doc library/lac/publications/CWH-Wellness%20Promotion and%20 Chronic Disease Prevention Initiatives.pdf
- Reports of Interest http://www.acmha.org/reports of interest.shtml

SUMMARY

The information and materials provided in this guide will continue to be updated and disseminated for use as the movement to ROSC and national health care solidifies policies and provides further guidance to stakeholders, providers, and policymakers vested in the substance use disorders field. As this evolution occurs, you may be just beginning to conceptualize ROSC for your community, while others are tackling implementation issues and beyond. Regardless of your stage in the planning and implementation process of ROSC, please use this resource guide as a tool to encourage discussion and strengthen the infrastructure of ROSC in your community.

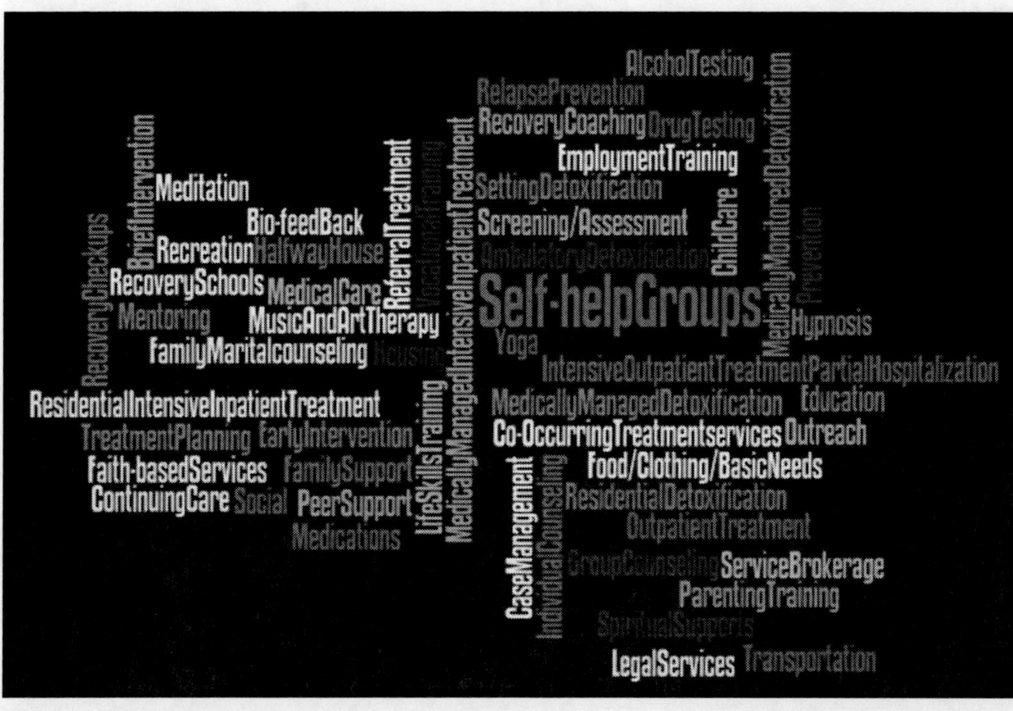

INDEX

C

J

L

M

Q

R

S

T